SIRTFOOD DIET

{Sirtfood easy and delicious recipes meal plan on how to burn fat and eat your way to a rapid weight loss and a longer healthy lifestyle}

2020

By

Harrison Cox

TABLE OF CONTENTS

PREFACE...1

INTRODUCTION 4

CHAPTER ONE: WHAT ARE SIRTFOODS? 7

CHAPTER TWO: FIGHTING FAT 24

CHAPTER THREE: MASTERS OF MUSCLE IN SIRTFOOD DIET...32

CHAPTER FOUR: WELL-BEING WONDERS IN SIRTFOOD 38

CHAPTER FIVE: SIRTFOODS 41

CHAPTER SIX: SIRTFOODS AROUND THE GLOBE 46

CHAPTER SEVEN: BUILDING A DIET THAT WORKS FOR YOU 53

CHAPTER EIGHT: TOP TWENTY SIRTFOODS DIET 65

CHAPTER NINE: PHASE 1: 7 POUNDS IN SEVEN DAYS....81

CHAPTER TEN: PHASE 2: MAINTENANCE 90

CHAPTER ELEVEN: SIRTFOODS FOR LIFE 97

CHAPTER TWELVE: SIRTFOODS FOR ALL...................... 113

CHAPTER THIRTEEN: SOCIAL EFFECTS ON OBESITY IN SIRTFOOD DIET 120

CHAPTER FOURTEEN: PSYCHOSOCIAL OUTCOMES OF OBESITY 131

CHAPTER FIFTEEN: FREQUENTLY ASKED QUESTIONS.. 143

CHAPTER SIXTEEN: RECIPES 153

REFERENCES 183

PREFACE

Nutrition assumes a key essential role in the achievement or disappointment of our day by day fights with the lump, from how we fuel our bodies and the food decisions we make to the bit sizes we serve. Everything appears sound system guidelines or advanced science, however consider the possibility that I let you know there was a simpler method to get in shape and be healthy.

I hate the word diet, as it conveys contrary implications for such a large number of individuals. The majority of my customers loathe the word as well. It causes them to feel like they've been given a life sentence to eat just exhausting and unacceptable dinners that will make them tumble off the wagon inside seven days! So why seize the chance to compose the foreword for The Sirtfood Diet? Why have I acquainted it with my customers to follow? My answer is very basic: It is not the same as each other diet that has preceded it. It is a totally different method of eating that brings phenomenal advantages for everybody.

I needed to show signs of improvement comprehension of how they functioned. I needed to realize things like: What were their impacts on the body? What sort of results was attainable? Did the guarantees they made just have momentary accomplishment with long haul disappointment? As I would see it, diets that advance weight reduction at the expense of your prosperity or power you to deny yourself of the nourishments you appreciate eating ought to be kept away from no matter what. Those kinds of dinner plans will just set you up for disappointment. My customers lack the capacity to deal with them. Some are high-genius le people who are continually under the investigation of the media spotlight. What they look like is given more significance and consideration than if they are cheerful and healthy. From exhausting professions and execution timetables to occupied day by day life, nutrition ought to not negatively affect any feature of life. It should just supplement and improve it.

They have a powerful enthusiasm for spreading the message of logically sponsored, precise nutrition, about how our cutting edge wellbeing troubles can be adjusted with the food we eat.

Despite that we could simply get the correct messages free from all the nutrition commotion, we might converse and stop the corpulence and sick wellbeing that plague us.

What's additionally phenomenal about the Sirtfood Diet is that it is a diet for food darlings. Such a large number of weight reduction and healthy-eating messages are separated from reality. You can't anticipate that individuals should eat the manner in which you recommend as long as possible Despite that it implies living in dietary hardship. The Sirtfood Diet turns this on its head. The advantages are all from eating tasty tasting food and not from what you are not eating. The more incredible tasting food you eat, the more advantages you see. It's the reason my customers love it! It additionally urges us to revive that lost relationship of appreciating eating times.

Contingent upon what your day by day life involves, regardless of whether it's dealing with a film set, being on a show world visit, or running a bustling family, the organization you keep bonds you as a family. Dinners are an occasion where everybody gets together to appreciate each other's conversation. With the Sirtfood Diet, this should effortlessly be possible.

Knowing the nourishments you are eating is supporting your prosperity. The plans are handy and easy to follow, while continually creating luscious suppers. There's genuine fulfillment in observing void plates and everybody content toward the finish of a dinner.

The word diet in the title of this book may nearly be an insult. This isn't a diet in the customary sense yet a method of eating forever. It's for each and every individual who needs to place their body into a more advantageous state and feel their best while as yet getting a charge out of life and their food. It's for individuals who need to see enormous contrasts from little changes and for the individuals who need weight reduction that keeps going without going through hours in the rec center or starving themselves.

I've encountered firsthand these amazing advantages. I have gone from saying I could never stop eating so much junk food to failing to eat some other way. Presently it's your opportunity to encounter and appreciate it as well!

INTRODUCTION

Susan felt her world deteriorate when she heard the word come out of her essential consideration doctor's mouth. This year, 2014, was planned to be her year. At just forty-one she had given up work two or three months sooner and was enthusiastically organizing her next life encounters.

In what could have graced Hollywood assessment content, she had as of late been united with her underlying life friend, Michael, ensuing to being isolated for quite a while. They would before their since a long time ago marry. By then she was told she had chest threatening development. . . .

Fortunately, the treatment was a triumph; anyway the responses of the chemotherapy brought about huge harm.

During the time Susan had reliably struggled with her weight and endeavored each diet design going, just to recuperate the weight notwithstanding even more each time. Nevertheless, directly she fundamentally didn't feel much improved. She felt "cumbersome, significant, and languid." She fell into a case of comfort eating, and the least troublesome of activities that she used to acknowledge, for instance, going out for a walk, needed to need to complete a significant distance race. Inside basically an issue of months Susan had expanded 20 pounds.

The expert by then instructed her that she would be on anticancer medication for the accompanying ten years. It was the standard calm called tamoxifen, prominent for causing weight expansion and lethargy.

She confronted the possibility of gulping a tablet consistently to fight off disease however to the detriment of her imperativeness and liking herself.

In any case, Susan was resolved not to let it beat her. Her presently spouse, Rannoch, the stone close by, was a diet cynic. Yet, having found out about another weight-loss diet dependent on the intensity of eating regular plant nourishments that flaunted huge prosperity benefits, he felt there was nothing to lose. Together, they set out upon the Sirtfood Diet. Inside the rest a month and a half, Susan shed 20 pounds. Rannoch himself had shed 12 pounds regardless of not conveying a lot of overabundance weight in the first place. This was a significant discovery for Susan; yet much progressively significant was the change by the way she felt. Her vitality levels took off and her get- up-and-go returned. The need to comfort eats vanished and lousy nourishment lost its intrigue. She had returned to her typical exercises once more, and as time passes she felt good and better. In Susan's words, "It is perhaps the best thing we have ever done; it's the best we have both felt in years. This isn't a diet in the standard sense, however a method of eating forever. I don't feel the reactions of the drug now, and I never need to stress over 'dieting' again."

Of the countless individuals who will follow advanced diets this year, under 1 percent will accomplish lasting weight loss.1 not just do they neglect to have any kind of effect in the clash of the lump, however they don't do anything to check the tidal wave of interminable ailment that has inundated current society.

We might be living longer yet we are not living more beneficial. Amazingly, through the span of a unimportant ten years, the measure of time we spend in sick wellbeing has multiplied from 20 to 40 percent. It implies we presently go through right around thirty-two years of our lives in unexpected frailty. Simply take a gander at the details. At this moment, one of every ten has diabetes and another three are very nearly getting it.

Two out of each five individuals will be determined to have malignant growth at some phase in their lives. On the off chance that you see three ladies beyond forty one years old, of them will have an osteoporotic break. What's more, in the normal time it takes you to peruse a solitary page of this book, another instance of Alzheimer's will create and somebody will kick the bucket of coronary illness—and that is in the United States alone.

Hence, "dieting" has never been our thing. That is, until we found Sirtfoods, a progressive new—and simple—approach to eat your approach to weight loss and astounding wellbeing.

CHAPTER ONE: WHAT ARE SIRTFOODS?

At the point when we cut back on calories, it makes a deficiency of vitality that actuates what is known as the "thin quality." This triggers a heap of positive changes. It places the body into a sort of endurance mode where it quits putting away fat and ordinary development forms are required to be postponed. Rather, the body directs its concentration toward consuming its stores of fat and turning on ground-breaking housekeeping qualities that fix and revive our phones, viably giving them a spring cleaning. The end result is weight loss and improved protection from ailment.

Be that as it may, the same number of dieters knows, cutting calories includes some significant downfalls. For the time being, the decrease in vitality admission incites hunger, crabbiness, weakness, and muscle loss. Longer-term calorie limitation makes our digestion deteriorate.

This is the ruin of all calorie-prohibitive diets and makes ready for the weight to return heaping on. It is consequently that 99 percent of dieters are destined to bomb over the long haul.

The entirety of this drove us to pose a major inquiry: is it some way or another conceivable to actuate our thin quality with all the incredible advantages that brings without expecting to adhere to extreme calorie limitation with each one of those disadvantages?

Enter Sirtfoods, a newfound gathering of marvel nourishments. Sirtfoods are especially wealthy in extraordinary supplements that, when we devour them, can enact similar thin qualities in our bodies that calorie limitation does. These qualities are known as sirtuins. They rest became known in a milestone concentrate in 2003 when specialists found that resveratrol, a compound found in red grape skin and red wine, drastically expanded the life length of yeast.2 Incredibly, resveratrol had a similar impact on life span as calorie limitation, yet this was accomplished without decreasing vitality consumption.

From that point forward investigations have demonstrated that resveratrol can expand life in worms, flies, fish, and even honeybees. And from mice to people, beginning time considers show resveratrol ensures against the unfriendly impacts of fatty, high-fat, and high-sugar diets; advances healthy maturing by postponing age-related maladies; and increments fitness generally it has been appeared to impersonate the impacts of calorie limitation and exercise.

With its rich resveratrol content, red wine was hailed as the first Sirtfood, clarifying the medical advantages connected to its utilization, and even why individuals who drink red wine increase less weight. However, this is just the start of the Sirtfood story.

With the disclosure of resveratrol, the universe of wellbeing research was on the cusp of something significant, and the pharmaceutical business burned through no time committing. Analysts started screening a large number of various synthetic substances for their capacity to initiate our sirtuin qualities. This uncovered various characteristic plant mixes, not only resveratrol, with huge sirtuin enacting properties. It was likewise found that a given food could contain an entire range of these plant mixes, which could work in show to both guide retention and boost that food's sirtuin-initiating impact. This had been one of the large riddles around resveratrol.

At the present time numerous investigations of sirtuin-initiating drugs are in progress for a huge number of ceaseless infections, just as the rest-ever FDA-affirmed preliminary to examine whether a medication can slow maturing.

As tempting as that may appear, if history has shown us anything, it's that we ought not to hold out a lot of trust in this pharmaceutical ambrosia. Consistently the pharmaceutical and wellbeing enterprises have attempted to copy the advantages of nourishments and diets through secluded medications and supplements. What's more, consistently it's missed the mark. Why sit tight ten or more years for the authorizing of these supposed miracle drugs, and the unavoidable reactions they bring, when right now we have all the amazing advantages accessible readily available through the food we eat?

So while the pharmaceutical business steadily seeks after a medication like enchantment shot, we need to retrain our attention on diet. For simultaneously those endeavors were in progress, the scene of nutritional research was additionally moving, bringing up some enormous issues of its own. Red wine to the other side, were there different nourishments with elevated levels of these extraordinary supplements fit for actuating our sirtuin qualities? What's more to it, assuming this is the case, what were their impacts on activating fat loss and battling illness?

NOT EVERY VEGETABLES AND FRUITS ARE DEVELOPED EQUALLY

Since 1986 two of the biggest nutritional examinations in US history have been attempted simultaneously by scientists at Harvard University: the Health Professionals Follow-Up Study, inspecting men's dietary propensities and wellbeing, and the Nurses' Health Study, exploring the equivalent for females. Drawing on this immense abundance of information, specialists investigated the connection between the dietary propensities for in excess of 124,000 individuals and changes in body weight over a twenty-four-year time span finishing off with 2011.6

They discovered something amazing. As a major aspect of a standard American diet, expending certain plant nourishments fought off weight gain, yet devouring others had no impact by any stretch of the imagination. What was the contrast between them?

Everything came down to whether the nourishments were wealthy in specific kinds of regular plant synthetic substances known as polyphenols. We about all will in general put on weight as we age, however expending higher measures of polyphenols had remarkable effect in forestalling this. When inspected in more prominent detail, just specific kinds of polyphenols stood apart as being powerful for keeping individuals thin, the scientists found.

Among those compelling were similar gatherings of normal plant synthetic substances that the pharmaceutical business was angrily attempting to transform into a marvel pill for their capacity to turn on our sirtuin qualities.

The end was significant: not all plant nourishments (counting products of the soil) are equivalent with regards to controlling our weight. Rather, we have to begin examining plant nourishments for their polyphenol substance, and afterward thusly explore the capacity of those polyphenols to turn on our "thin" sirtuin qualities. This is an extreme thought that contradicts the overarching doctrine of our occasions. The time has come to relinquish the nonexclusive, cover counsel that instructs us to eat two cups of products of the soil and a half cups of vegetables daily as a component of a fair diet. We need just check out us to perceive how little effect that has had.

With this move in judging how plant nourishments are beneficial for us, something different got obvious. The numerous nourishments that alleged wellbeing specialists cautioned us away from, for example, chocolate, espresso, and tea, are in reality so rich in sirtuin enacting polyphenols that they trump most products of the soil out there. How often do we scowl as we swallow our vegetables since we're informed that is the correct activity, possibly to feel remorseful on the off chance that we even glance at that after supper chocolate treat?

A definitive incongruity is that cocoa is perhaps the best food we might be eating. Its utilization has now been demonstrated to initiate sirtuin qualities, with different advantages for controlling body weight by consuming fat, lessening craving, and improving muscle function.7 and that is before we assess its large number of other medical advantages, a greater amount of which to come later.

In all out we have recognized twenty nourishments rich in polyphenols that have been appeared to actuate our sirtuin qualities, and together these structure the premise of the Sirtfood Diet. While the story began with red wine as the first Sirtfood, we presently realize these other nineteen nourishments either match or trump it for their sirtuin-initiating polyphenol content. Just as cocoa, these incorporate other notable and much-appreciated nourishments, for example, additional virgin olive oil, red onions, garlic, parsley, chilies, kale, strawberries, pecans, escapades, tofu, green tea, and even espresso. While every food has amazing wellbeing qualifications of its own, as we are going to see, the genuine enchantment happens when we consolidate these nourishments to make an entire diet.

A COMMON LINK AMONG THE WORLD'S HEALTHIEST DIETS

As we inquired about further, we found that the best wellsprings of Sirtfoods were found in the diets of those bragging the most minimal rates sickness and corpulence on the planet—from the Kuna American Indians, who seem insusceptible to hypertension and show strikingly low paces of stoutness, diabetes, malignant growth, and early demise, on account of a fabulously rich admission of the Sirtfood cocoa; to Okinawa, Japan, where a smorgasbord of Sirtfoods, smooth guts, and long life all go connected at the hip; to India, where the insatiable hunger for everything zesty, particularly the Sirtfood turmeric, has left disease afterward.

However, the diet is the jealousy of the remainder of the Western world, a customary Mediterranean diet, where the advantages of Sirtfoods genuinely stick out. Here heftiness basically doesn't win and constant sickness is the special case, not the standard. Additional virgin olive oil, wild verdant greens, nuts, berries, red wine, dates, and herbs are generally intense Sirtfoods and all components conspicuously in the local Mediterranean diet. The logical world has been left in wonderment considering the latest agreement that following a Mediterranean diet is more compelling than checking calories for weight loss, and more successful than pharmaceutical medications for halting disease.

This carries us to PREDIMED, a game-changing investigation of the Mediterranean diet, distributed in 2013. It was directed on right around 7,400 people at high danger of cardiovascular infection, and the outcomes were acceptable to the point that the preliminary was really halted ahead of schedule—after only five years.

The reason of PREDIMED was flawlessly straightforward. It asked what the distinction would be between a Mediterranean-style diet enhanced with either additional virgin olive oil or nuts (particularly pecans) and an increasingly regular cutting edge diet. Also, what a distinction it was. The adjustment in diet diminished the occurrence of cardiovascular sickness by around 30 percent, an outcome tranquilize organizations can just dream of. Upon further development, it was discovered that there was additionally a 30 percent fall in diabetes, alongside huge drops in ambition, upgrades in memory and cerebrum wellbeing, and a gigantic 40 percent decrease in weight, with remarkable fat loss particularly around the stomach region.

However at first analysts couldn't clarify what created these emotional advantages. Neither the measures of calories, fats, and sugars eaten—the commonplace estimates used to survey the food we eat—nor did physical action levels contrast between the gatherings to clarify the discoveries. There must be something different going on.

At that point the aha second struck. Both additional virgin olive oil and pecans stand apart for their outstanding substance of sirtuin-actuating polyphenols. Basically, by adding these in critical adds up to an ordinary Mediterranean diet, what the scientists had accidentally made was a superrich Sirtfood diet, and they found that it conveyed stunning outcomes.

So scientists breaking down PREDIMED thought of an astute speculation. In the event that it is the polyphenols that at last issue, they considered, at that point the individuals who ate the vast majority of them would encounter their aggregate advantages by living the longest.

So they ran the details, and the outcomes were faltering. Over only five years, the individuals who devoured the most significant levels of polyphenols had 37 percent less passing's contrasted with the individuals who ate the least.10 Intriguingly, this is twofold the decrease in mortality that treatment with the most ordinarily recommended blockbuster statin drugs is found to bring. At last we had the clarification for the marvelous advantages this investigation watched, and it was more impressive than any medication in presence.

The analysts likewise noted something different of significance. While numerous examinations have recently discovered that individual Sirtfoods present great medical advantages, they were never significant enough to really expand life. PREDIMED was the remainder of its sort. The thing that matters was that it took a gander at an example of nourishments as opposed to a solitary food.

Various nourishments give distinctive sirtuin-enacting polyphenols, which work in concordance to deliver a significantly more remarkable result than any single food can. This left us with an enthusiastic end.

Genuine wellbeing isn't procured through one single supplement or even one "wonder food." What you need is an entire diet loaded up with a mix of Sirtfoods all working in cooperative energy. What's more, this is the thing that prompted the production of the Sirtfood Diet.

THE SIRTFOOD STUDY

A tiny bit at a time, we had sorted out all the perceptions from customary societies and discoveries from major logical examinations, coming full circle in PREDIMED, perhaps the best investigation of diet at any point directed. Be that as it may, even the discoveries of PREDIMED, in the same way as other wellbeing advancements, came through possibility. It never set out to plan and tests a diet of Sirtfoods. It was just later that science found this was adequately what PREDIMED had done.

This implied there were as yet numerous Sirtfoods the diet had excluded that could have expanded its colossal advantages significantly further.

Furthermore, all the exploration to date had set up the advantages for long haul weight the board and diminishing ailment. Be that as it may, we despite everything didn't have the foggiest idea how rapidly those advantages for body weight and prosperity could be figured it out. We as a whole need to ensure our future wellbeing yet would prefer us not to look and feel great in the present time and place as well?

To respond to these inquiries, we required an intentionally led Sirtfood Diet intercession that incorporated every one of the twenty of the most remarkable Sirtfoods for which we could accumulate prior estimations of the outcomes. So we set out on our very own pilot investigation. Settled in the core of London, England, is KX, one of Europe's generally looked for after wellbeing and wellness focuses. What makes KX the ideal spot to test the impacts of the Sirtfood Diet is that it has its own café, which gave us the open door to plan the diet, however to breathe life into it and test it on the wellness place's individuals.

Our dispatch was clear. For seven days straight, individuals would follow our deliberately built Sirtfood Diet and we would fastidiously keep tabs on their development from start to finish, estimating their weight, yet in addition observing changes in their body synthesis, which implied checking how the diet influenced the degrees of fat and muscle in the body. Afterward, we included metabolic measures, to see the impacts of the diet on levels of sugar (glucose) and fats (like triglycerides and cholesterol) in the blood.

The rest three days were the most extreme, with food consumption limited to 1,000 calories for every day. As a result, this resembles a gentle quick, which is significant in light of the fact that the let vitality admission turns down development flags in the body and urges it to begin getting old trash out of cells (a procedure known as autophagy) and launch fat consuming. In any case, dissimilar to mainstream fasting diets, this quick was gentle and brief, making it considerably more maintainable, as demonstrated by the investigation's astoundingly high 97.5 percent adherence rate. Additionally, we needed to research the distinctions that adding Sirtfoods made to the ordinary ruins experienced with fasting diets. Also, as we were soon to discover, they were emotional.

Our essential objective was to have a major effect to the fat-consuming impacts of this mellow calorie limitation by pressing the diet loaded with Sirtfoods. This was accomplished by putting together the everyday diet with respect to three Sirtfood-rich green juices and one Sirtfood-rich dinner.

For the last four days of our program at KX, calories were expanded to 1,500 every day. Viably this was just a mellow calorie deficiency, however enough to keep development signals turned down and fat-consuming signs turned. Significantly, that 1,500-calorie diet was jam-pressed with Sirtfoods, comprising of two Sirtfood-rich green juices and two Sirtfood-rich dinners every day.

THE REMARKABLE RESULTS

The Sirtfood Diet was tried by forty and finished by thirty-nine individuals at KX. Of these thirty-nine, two in the preliminary were hefty, fifteen were overweight, and twenty-two had an ordinary/healthy weight list (BMI).

The investigation had a genuinely even sexual orientation split, with twenty-one ladies and eighteen men. Being individuals from a fitness center, before they began they were bound to practice and know about healthy eating than everyone.

A stunt of numerous diets is to utilize an intensely overweight and unhealthy example of individuals to show the advantages, as very still they get thinner the fastest and most drastically, basically of bother up the diet results. Our rationale was the inverse: on the off chance that we acquired great outcomes with this generally healthy gathering, it would set the base benchmark of what was feasible.

The outcomes far surpassed our effectively elevated standards. Results were reliable and amazing: a normal 7 pounds of weight loss in seven days in the wake of representing muscle gain.

As though that weren't commendable enough, we saw something different considerably progressively great, which the sort of weight loss was. Regularly, when individuals get in shape, they will lose some fat yet they will likewise lose some muscle—this is not all bad with regards to dieting. We were shocked to find the inverse. Our members either kept up their muscle or really picked up muscle. As we will find out later in the book, this is an in nitely progressively ideal kind of weight loss, and an extraordinary element of the Sirtfood Diet.

No member neglected to see enhancements in body synthesis. What's more, recall, the entirety of this was accomplished without dietary hardship or exhausting activity regimens.

This is what we found:

- Participants accomplished sensational and fast outcomes, losing a normal of 7 pounds in seven days
- Weight loss was generally recognizable around the stomach zone.

- Rather than being lost, bulk was either kept up or expanded

- Participants once in a while felt hungry

- Participants felt an expanded feeling of imperativeness and prosperity.

- Participants revealed looking better and more beneficial.

A DIET IN THE REAL WORLD

It's one thing to get incredible outcomes following a diet in a controlled situation where all the food is expertly made and given, and nutrition specialists are close by to answer any questions. It's something different by and large when individuals are left to fight for themselves with nothing more to help them than can be found in the pages of this very book. In any case, it was these reports that truly took our breath away. A diet that can so intensely advance fat loss and improve body creation while turbocharging vitality levels and prosperity has numerous valuable applications. In a little while, several tributes had poured in. From brandishing hotshots who were title holders and Olympic gold medalists to TV characters and models to the greatest names in showbiz, in addition to the fact that they were tailing it and adhering to it, yet they were raving about it.

Readers were crushing the 7 pounds in seven days weight loss we'd found in our preliminary, demonstrating our theory that our as of now t and healthy examination populace was disparaging the advantages. The most extreme weight loss we have seen to date was with a columnist and diet skeptic who set out to freely test the program's benefits. Rather than castigating it, he shed 14 pounds in the principal week. Safe to state he presently joins the companions of changes over. Away from the scales, others revealed similarly amazing outcomes through inches lost around the midriff. Furthermore, the best part is that the weight was remaining off, with the outcomes just improving throughout the months.

As fabulous as this input might have been, for us as nutritional medication advisors who spend significant time in turning around and forestalling malady, there was something that roused us much more: the individual stories that, much the same as Susan's toward the beginning of this part, were out and out life-evolving.

There was Robert, who had languished sadness over years. He shed 10 pounds in only fourteen days however was unquestionably progressively charmed with the lifting of his discouraged state of mind, to such an extent that he was "cherishing life" again. Melanie was in horrendous torment with lupus. Five weeks in, she was down 11.5 pounds, yet significantly more significant, her a throbbing painfulness had evaporated. Actually, she had no lupus side effects by any means. Feeling astounding, she no longer needed to go to her master; there was nothing to treat. Also, Linda, who was down a mind boggling 50 pounds following three months, switched her declining diabetes and had the vitality again to appreciate life once more.

This is only a sample of the numerous moving stories that have come in. Coronary illness has switched. Menopause side effects have stopped. Crabby gut conditions have vanished. Without precedent for years individuals were resting soundly once more. One puzzled ophthalmologist even reached us with the news that after only seven days on the Sirtfood Diet, her patient's incessant sclera staining had completely turned around and was currently flawless white once more. She even sent photographs for evidence.

HOW THE SIRTFOOD DIET WILL WORK FOR YOU

The sheer expansiveness of advantages that individuals have encountered has been a disclosure; all accomplished by just putting together their diet with respect to open and moderate nourishments that a great many people as of now appreciate eating. What's more, that is all the Sirtfood Diet requires. It's tied in with receiving the rewards of ordinary nourishments that we were constantly intended to eat, yet in the correct amounts and the correct mixes to give us the body structure and prosperity we as a whole so beyond all doubt need, and that can at last transform us.

It doesn't expect you to perform extreme calorie limitation, nor does it request tiring activity regimens (despite the fact that, obviously, remaining commonly dynamic is something to be thankful for). What's more, the main bit of gear you'll require is a juicer. In addition, not at all like each other diet out there that centers on what you ought to prohibit, the Sirtfood Diet centers around what you ought to incorporate. To summarize everything, the Sirtfood Diet will support you.

- lose weight by consuming fat, not muscle

- Burn fat, particularly from the stomach zone, to fuel better wellbeing

- Prime your body for long haul weight-loss achievement

- look and feel much improved and have more vitality

- Avoid suffering serious calorie limitation or outrageous yearning

- Be liberated from exhausting activity routine

- live a more extended, more beneficial, ailment free life

THE SCIENCE OF SIRTUINS

What makes the Sirtfood Diet so amazing is its capacity to turn on an old group of qualities that exists in every one of us. The name for this group of qualities is sirtuin. Sirtuins are exceptional on the grounds that they coordinate procedures profound inside our cells that impact such significant things as our capacity to consume fat, our helplessness—or not—too illness, and at last even our life range. So significant is the impact of sirtuins that they are currently alluded to as "ace metabolic regulators."[1] fundamentally, precisely what anybody needing to shed a few pounds and carry on with a long and healthy life would need to be accountable for?

OF MICE AND MEN

Justifiably, sirtuins have become the subject of exceptional logical research lately. The first sirtuin was found in 1984 in yeast, and intrigue truly took off through the span of the following three decades when it was uncovered that sirtuin actuation builds life length, first in yeast, and afterward as far as possible up to mice.

Why the energy? Since from yeast to people and everything in the middle of, the crucial standards of cell digestion are almost indistinguishable. On the off chance that you can control something as small as sprouting yeast and see an advantage, at that point rehash it in higher creatures, for example, mice, the potential exists for similar advantages to be acknowledged in people.

AN APPETITE FOR FASTING

The lifelong limitation of food admission has reliably been appeared to expand the life hope of lower creatures and mammals.

This striking Findings is the reason for the act of caloric limitation among certain individuals, where every day calorie admission is diminished by around 20 to 30 percent, just as its advanced branch, irregular fasting, which has become an effective weight-loss diet, put on the map by any semblance of the 5:2 diet, or Fast Diet.

While we despite everything anticipate evidence of expanded life length for people from these practices, there is verification of advantages for what we may term "wellbeing range"— constant illnesses drop and fat begins to liquefy away.

In any case, let's face it, regardless of how huge the advantages, fasting week in, week out, is a tiresome business that the greater parts of us aren't happy to read. Regardless of whether we do, a large portion of us can't adhere to it.

On this there are downsides to fasting, particularly when we tail it long haul. In the presentation we referenced the reactions of yearning, fractiousness, weariness, muscle loss, and digestion lull. Yet, also, progressing fasting regimens could put us in danger of malnutrition, influencing our prosperity because of a brought down admission of basic supplements.

Fasting regimens are additionally completely inadmissible for huge extents of the populace, for example, youngsters, ladies during pregnancy, and potentially the old. While there are plainly settled advantages to fasting, it's not the enchantment slug we might want it to be. It made them ask, is this actually the manner in which nature planned for us to be dainty and healthy? Unquestionably there's a superior way. . . .

Our advancement came when we found that the significant advantages from caloric limitation and fasting were intervened through enactment of our old sirtuin genes to more readily get this, it may be useful to consider sirtuins as the watchmen at the junction between vitality status and life span. What they do there is react to stresses.

At the point when vitality is hard to come by, precisely as we see in caloric limitation, there is an expansion in weight on our cells. This is detected by the sirtuins, which at that point get turned on and communicate a group of stars of ground-breaking signals that fundamentally modify the manner in which cells act. Sirtuins increase our digestion, increment the effectiveness of our muscles, switch on fat consuming, diminish in ambition, and fix any harm in our cells. As a result, sirtuins make us fitter, more slender, and more beneficial.

A ZEAL FOR EXERCISE

It's not simply caloric limitation and fasting that initiate sirtuins; practice does too.6 simply like in fasting, sirtuins coordinate the significant advantages of activity. Be that as it may, while we are urged to take part in normal moderate exercise for its large number of advantages, it isn't the methods through which we are intended to center our weight-loss endeavors.

Research shows that the human body has advanced approaches to normally alter and decrease the measure of vitality we use when we work out, 7 implying that with the goal for exercise to be compelling weight-loss mediation, we have to submit considerable time and difficult exertion. That difficult exercise regimens are the manner in which nature proposed us to keep up a healthy weight is considerably increasingly questionable considering research presently recommending that a lot of activity can be hurtful—debilitating our insusceptible frameworks, harming the heart, and adding to early death.

ENTER SIRTFOODS

So far we have found that in the event that we need to get more fit and be healthy, the key is to actuate our sirtuin qualities. As of not long ago the two realized approaches to accomplish this have been fasting and exercise. Oh, the sums required for fruitful weight loss accompany their downsides, and for a large portion of us are just inconsistent with how we live in the twenty-first century.

Luckily, there is a newfound, noteworthy method for actuating our sirtuin qualities in the most ideal manner: Sirtfoods.

As we will before long learn, these are the marvel nourishments especially wealthy in explicit characteristic plant synthetic compounds that have the ability to address our sirtuin qualities, turning them on. Fundamentally they impersonate the impacts of fasting and practice and in doing so bring astounding advantages of consuming fat, building muscle, and boosting wellbeing, which were beforehand unreachable.

RUNDOWN

- Each of us has an old group of qualities called sirtuins.

- Sirtuins are ace metabolic controllers that control our capacity to consume fat and remain healthy.

- Sirtuins go about as vitality sensors inside our cells, and get actuated when a lack of vitality is recognized.

- Fasting and exercise both initiate our sirtuin qualities, yet can be difficult to adhere to and even have downsides.

- There is another earth shattering approach to enact our sirtuin qualities.

CHAPTER TWO: FIGHTING FAT

One of the emotional Discoveries from our pilot investigation of the Sirtfood Diet was not simply the measure of weight the members lost, which was amazing enough — it was the sort of weight loss that truly got us energized. What caught our eye was the way that numerous individuals were getting in shape without losing any muscle. Actually, it was normal to see individuals gain muscle.

This left us with an inevitable end: fat was simply dissolving endlessly.

Regularly, accomplishing noteworthy fat loss requires an impressive penance, either seriously decreasing calories or taking part in superhuman degrees of activity, or both. However, as opposed to that, our members either kept up or diminished their activity levels, and didn't report feeling especially eager. Indeed, some even attempted to eat all the food that was accommodated them. How is this even conceivable? It's just when we comprehend what befalls our fat cells when sirtuin action is expanded that we can start to understand these noteworthy discoveries.

LEAN QUALITIES

Mice that have been hereditarily built to have elevated levels of SIRT1, the sirtuin quality that drives fat loss, are more slender and all the more metabolically dynamic, while mice lacking SIRT1 are fatter and have progressively metabolic disease.2 when we see people; levels of SIRT1 have been seen as particularly

Lower in the muscle versus fat of stout individuals than their healthy-weight partners. Conversely, individuals with expanded SIRT1 quality action are less fatty and increasingly impervious to weight gain.

Stack all that up and you begin to get a feeling of exactly how significant sirtuins are for deciding if we remain lean or get fat, and why by expanding sirtuin action you can accomplish such astounding outcomes. This is on the grounds that through sirtuins we get benefits on numerous levels, beginning at the very base, all things considered, and the qualities that control weight gain.

To all the more likely get this, we have to dig further into what occurs in our cells that makes us put on weight.

CONTEXTUAL ANALYSIS

Kate is a housewife in her mid-thirties and mother to two little youngsters. With a muscle versus fat estimation of in excess of 25 percent, she was classed as "Satisfactory" as far as the measure of fat put away in her body, yet was miserable that she was all the while conveying those additional couple of pregnancy pounds around the center. Regardless of being very dynamic—practicing in the rec center when she could and being continually on her feet with two vitality filled youngsters to care for—her weight didn't move. Diet-wise she had consistently attempted to eat steadily, and expressed that, on the off chance that anything, she ate excessively little rather than something over the top, with it not being phenomenal for her to skirt a feast to guarantee the kids were cared for.

The straightforwardness and comfort of the Sirtfood Diet made it ideal for her to give it a shot, and she accomplished fabulous outcomes. Before a week's over Kate was down 6 pounds 8 ounces on the scales and had increased 1 pound in muscle for a net fat loss of 7 pounds 8 ounces. Her muscle to fat ratio was presently 22 percent, placing her in the "t" runs that she so wanted.

FAT BUSTING

We will clarify this as far as a Hollywood medication ring lm.

The fooding of the avenues with drugs is the fooding of our body with fat. The medication pushers on the traffic intersections are what might be compared to the responses in our body that sell weight gain. Be that as it may, truly, they are just the low-level hooligans. Behind everything is the genuine miscreant engineering the entire activity, coordinating each arrangement the vendors make. In our lm, this scalawag is called PPAR-γ (peroxisome proliferator-enacted receptor-γ). PPAR-γ organizes the fat addition process by turning on the qualities that are expected to begin orchestrating and putting away fat. To stop the proliferation of fat, you should cut the flexibly. Stop PPAR-γ, and you successfully stop fat increase. Enter our legend, SIRT1, who ascends to cut down the scoundrel. With the miscreant safely bolted up, there is nobody to call the shots and the entire fat increase association disintegrates. With the action of PPAR-γ stopped, SIRT1 moves its considerations to "cleaning the lanes." In addition to the fact that this is finished by closing down the creation and capacity of fat, as we've seen, however it really changes our digestion so we begin freeing the assemblage of overabundance fat.

Much the same as each great wrongdoing battling saint, SIRT1 has a sidekick, a key controller in our cells known as PGC-1α. This capably invigorates the production of what are known as mitochondria. These are the minuscule vitality manufacturing plants that exist inside every one of our phones—the force the body. The more mitochondria we have, the more vitality we can deliver. In any case, not exclusively does PGC-1α advance more mitochondria; it additionally urges them to consume fat as the fuel of decision to make the vitality. So from one viewpoint fat stockpiling is blocked, and on the other fat consuming is expanded.

CONTEXTUAL INVESTIGATION

Linda is a night-move laborer in her fries. Essentially overweight for a long time, in the same way as other she had attempted all the most recent diets, however without progress. At that point two years back the inescapable occurred: Linda was determined to have type 2 diabetes. She was put on the mainstream diabetes medicate metformin, yet her glucose levels kept on falling apart to where she was near the precarious edge of requiring treatment with insulin too. Frantic to not capitulate to a lifetime of different day by day infusions, Linda requested The Sirtfood Diet in the wake of hearing how others had lost such a great amount of weight on it.

N only multi week, Linda lost a stunning 13 pounds. Twelve weeks in, her weight had dropped by an amazing 50 pounds, reflected in her BMI, which was presently somewhere near an unimaginable seven focuses. Even more striking was the way this was accomplished with no activity at all, simply the intensity of Sirtfoods. Concerning renouncing all the things that Linda cherished? Nothing could be further from reality, as she was glad to call attention to, "I anticipate my chocolate and red wine— Pinot Noir is beautiful. It's simply being reasonable with the terrible stuff and wolfing down the great."

Far better news was to come at her half year diabetic test: unimaginably, her glucose levels were currently typical. Linda had not just ended the disintegration of her illness, she had turned around it. With Sirtfoods now settled as a major aspect of her regular day to day existence, and with her vitality levels soaring, Linda is presently prepared to set out on some activity as well, making ready for additional weight loss and a future liberated from diabetes.

WAT OR BAT?

So far we've taken a gander at the impacts of SIRT1 on fat loss on a notable sort of fat called white fat tissue (WAT).

This is the kind of fat related with weight gain. It has practical experience away and extension, is unpleasantly difficult, and secretes a large group of inflammatory synthetic compounds that oppose fat consuming and support further fat aggregation, making us overweight and corpulent. This is the reason weight gain frequently begins gradually yet can snowball so rapidly.

Be that as it may, there is another charming edge to the sirtuin story, including a lesser known sort of fat, earthy colored fat tissue (BAT), which carries on in an unexpected way. In complete differentiation to white fat tissue, BAT is advantageous to us and needs to get spent. Earthy colored fat tissue really encourages us exhaust vitality and has advanced in well evolved creatures to permit them to disperse a lot of vitality as warmth.

This is known as a thermo genic impact and is basic to little warm blooded creatures to assist them with getting by in chilly temperatures. In people, babies likewise have huge measures of earthy colored fat tissue, in spite of the fact that it diminishes not long after birth, leaving littler sums in grown-ups.

Here is the place SIRT1 actuation accomplishes something really astounding. It turns on qualities in our white fat tissue with the goal that it transforms and assumes the properties of earthy colored fat tissue in what is known as a "sautéing effect."8 That implies our fat stores begin to act in an out and out various way—rather than putting away vitality, they begin to assemble it for removal.

As should be obvious, sirtuin actuation has strong direct activity on fat cells, urging fat to soften away. However, it doesn't end there. Sirtuins likewise decidedly impact the most important hormones associated with weight control.

Sirtuin actuation improves insulin action. This assists with decreasing insulin obstruction—the powerlessness of our cells to react appropriately to insulin—which is intensely involved in weight gain. SIRT1 likewise improves the discharge and action of our thyroid hormones, which share many covering jobs in boosting our digestion and at last the rate at which we copy fat.

HUNGER CONTROL

There was one thing we were unable to fold our heads over in our pilot study: in spite of a decrease in calories, members didn't generally get eager. Indeed, a few people attempted to eat all the food gave.

One of the huge points of interest of the Sirtfood Diet is that we can accomplish extraordinary advantages without the requirement for long haul calorie limitation. The very rest seven day stretch of the diet is the hyper-achievement stage, where we join moderate fasting with a plenitude of ground-breaking Sirtfoods for a twofold hit to fat. What's more, similarly as with all fasting regimens, we anticipated a few reports of appetite here. In any case, we got completely none!

As we trawled through research, we found the appropriate response. It's everything because of the body's first craving controlling hormone, leptin, nicknamed the "satiety hormone." When we eat, leptin expands, motioning to a piece of the mind considered the nerve center that represses hunger. Alternately, when we quick, leptin motioning to the cerebrum diminishes, causing us to feel hungry. So significant is leptin in directing hunger that early expectations were that it could be regulated as an "enchantment projectile" to treat stoutness. Be that as it may, that fantasy was broken with the acknowledgment that the metabolic brokenness that happens in stoutness really causes leptin to quit working appropriately. In weight, not exclusively is the measure of leptin that can get into the mind decreased yet the nerve center additionally becomes desensitized to its activities.

This is known as leptin opposition: the leptin is there however no longer works appropriately. Consequently for some, overweight people, despite the fact that they eat enough, the mind keeps on speculation they are starved and flags for them to keep on searching out food.

The consequence of this is while the degree of leptin in the blood is significant for managing hunger, what is undeniably increasingly significant is its amount arrives at the mind and can affect the nerve center. This is the place Sirtfoods sparkle.

New proof shows that the supplements found in Sirtfoods have one of a kind advantages for turning around leptin opposition. This is through both expanding the vehicle of leptin to the mind and expanding the affectability of the nerve center to lepton's activities. So back to our unique inquiry: for what reason don't individuals feel hungry on the Sirtfood Diet? In spite of a drop in leptin levels in the blood during the gentle quick, which would regularly expand hunger, including Sirtfoods into the diet causes leptin motioning to turn out to be progressively productive, bringing about improved craving guideline.

As we will see later, Sirtfoods additionally effects affect our taste places, which means we get considerably more joy and fulfillment from our food and don't along these lines fall into the snare of gorging to feel fulfilled.

In any event, for the most committed dieters, sirtuins are probably going to be a fresh out of the plastic new idea. However focusing on sirtuins, the ace controllers of our digestion, is the foundation of any fruitful weight-loss diet. Shockingly, the very idea of our advanced society, with plenteous food and stationary lifestyles, makes an ideal tempest for turning off our sirtuin movement, and we see the aftermath of this overall us.

Fortunately now we recognize what sirtuins are, the manner by which they control fat stockpiling and advance fat consuming, and generally significant, how to turn them on. What's more, with this progressive discovery, finally the response to viable and supported weight loss is yours for the taking.

SYNOPSIS

- Fat liquefies away on the Sirtfood Diet. This is on the grounds that sirtuins have the ability to decide if we remain lean or get fat.

- Activating SIRT1 represses PPAR-γ, obstructing the creation and capacity of fat.

- Activating SIRT1 additionally turns on PGC-1, which makes more vitality production lines in our cells and expands fat consuming.

- Activating SIRT1 even gets our fat cells that spend significant time in vitality stockpiling to carry on distinctively and begin discarding vitality.

You are probably not going to feel hungry on the Sirtfood Diet since it assists with controlling craving in the mind.

CHAPTER THREE: MASTERS OF MUSCLE IN SIRTFOOD DIET

A striking finding from our pilot preliminary that truly got us fascinated was that the bulk of the members didn't drop; truth be told, it expanded, on normal by a little more than 1 pound. While it was not unexpected to see weight loss of 7 beats on the scales, we additionally observed something intriguing happening. For right around 66% of our members, the losses on the scales at first showed up more frustrating than this, yet still exceptionally amazing, with a weight loss of a little more than 5 pounds.

Be that as it may, when body organization tests were performed, we were stunned. Bulk was not simply kept up in these members, it had expanded. The normal muscle gain for this gathering was just about 2 pounds, giving what is known as a "muscle put on balanced weight loss" of 7 pounds.

This was totally startling and as a glaring difference to what regularly occurs on weight-loss diets; where individuals lose some fat however they additionally lose muscle. It's the great exchange off for any diet that limits calories: you kiss muscle farewell just as fat. This isn't at all amazing when you consider that when we deny the assemblage of vitality, cells move from growth mode to endurance mode and will utilize the protein from muscle for fuel.

WHAT'S SO ACCEPTABLE ABOUT LOOKING AFTER MUSCLE?

So what's the serious deal? You may inquire. Right off the bat, it implies you'll look much better. Stripping ceaselessly fat, yet holding muscle prompts an increasingly attractive slender, conditioned, and athletic physical make-up. What's more, significantly progressively significant, you'll remain looking great. Skeletal muscle is the central point that represents our body's day by day vitality use. This implies the more muscle you have, the more vitality you consume, in any event, while resting. This truly assists with supporting further weight loss and improves the probability of achievement in the long haul. As we presently know, with run of the mill dieting, weight loss originates from both fat loss and muscle loss, and with that we see a stamped decrease in the metabolic rate.

This prepares for weight recapture when progressively ordinary dietary patterns are continued. Be that as it may, by keeping hold of your bulk with Sirtfoods, you consume fatter with a negligible drop in metabolic rate. This gives the ideal establishment to long haul weight-loss achievement.

Also, bulk and capacity is an indicator of prosperity and healthy maturing, and keeping up muscle forestalls the advancement of ceaseless sicknesses, for example, diabetes and osteoporosis, just as keeping us portable into more seasoned age. Critically, it additionally seems to keep us more joyful, with researchers recommending that the way sirtuins keep up muscle even has benefits for pressure related clutters, including diminishing sadness.

All things considered, shedding pounds while securing muscle is a big deal and an in daily progressively great result it's a remarkable component of the Sirtfood Diet, and to more readily get this, we have to return to sirtuins and their incredible consequences for muscle. **SIRTUINS AND BULK**

There is a group of qualities in the body that go about as watchmen of our muscle and stop its breakdown when under pressure: the sirtuins.2 SIRT1 is an intense inhibitor of muscle breakdown. For whatever length of time that SIRT1 is initiated, in any event, when we are fasting, muscle breakdown is forestalled and we keep on consuming fat for fuel.

However, the advantages of SIRT1 don't end with protecting bulk. Sirtuins really work to build our skeletal muscle mass.3–5 to clarify how this wonder functions; we have to wander into the energizing universe of undifferentiated organisms. Our muscle contains an extraordinary kind of immature microorganism, called a satellite cell, which controls its growth and recovery. Satellite cells simply stay there unobtrusively more often than not, yet they are enacted when muscle gets harmed or focused.

This is the means by which our muscles get greater through exercises like weight preparing. SIRT1 is fundamental for enacting satellite cells, and without its action muscles are essentially littler on the grounds that they no longer have the ability to create or recover properly.6 Be that as it may, by expanding SIRT1 action, we give a lift to our satellite cells, which empowers muscle growth and recuperation.

SIRTFOODS AS OPPOSED TO FASTING

This leads us to an unavoidable issue: on the off chance that sirtuin enactment expands bulk, at that point for what reason do we lose muscle when we quick? All things considered, fasting enacts our sirtuin qualities also. What's more, in this lays one of the enormous disadvantages of fasting.

Hold on for us while we dive into how this functions. Not all skeletal muscle is made equivalent. We have two primary sorts, advantageously called type-1 and type-2. Type-1 muscle is utilized for longer-span exercises, while type-2 muscle is utilized for short eruptions of increasingly extreme movement. What's more, here's the place it gets captivating: fasting builds SIRT1 action just in type-1 muscle fibers, not in type-2.7 so type-1 muscle size is kept up and even perceptibly increments when we fast.8 tragically, in complete differentiation to what occurs in type-1 fibers during fasting, SIRT1 quickly decreases in type-2 fibers. This implies fat torching eases back, and rather muscle begins to separate to give fuel.

So fasting is a twofold edged blade for muscles, with our sort 2 fibers enduring a shot. Type- 2 fibers are what involve the greater part of our muscle definition. So despite the fact that our sort 1 fiber mass builds, we despite everything see a general huge loss of muscle with fasting. In the event that we could stop the breakdown, it would make us look great stylishly as well as help advance further fat loss. Also, the best approach to do this is to battle the drop in SIRT1 in type-2 muscle fiber achieved by fasting.

In an exquisite mice study, scientists at Harvard Clinical School put this under a magnifying glass, and indicated that by invigorating SIRT1 action in type-2 fibers during fasting, the signs for muscle breakdown were turned off and muscle loss didn't occur.9

The scientists at that point went above and beyond and tried the impacts of expanded SIRT1 action on muscle when the mice were taken care of as opposed to fasted, and found that it activated extremely quick muscle growth. Inside only seven days, muscle fibers with expanded degrees of SIRT1 action indicated a bewildering 20 percent expansion in weight.10

These foodings are fundamentally the same as the result of our Sirtfood Diet preliminary, however our investigation was milder essentially. By expanding SIRT1 action through eating a diet rich in Sirtfoods, most of members had no muscle loss — and for some, with it just being a moderate quick, bulk really expanded.

CONTEXTUAL ANALYSIS

David has earned notoriety for being one of the most skilled fighters on the planet, however in the heavyweight classification he frequently confronted adversaries who conveyed 20 to 40 pounds more muscle than he. Also, having been down and out for such a long time with a physical issue implied that he was conveying around 20 pounds more muscle versus fat than a world class confining hero this classification should.

What was essential to him for his arrival to the ring was to expand bulk while losing fat. A devoted advocate of plant-based diets, he wholeheartedly embraced the Sirtfood approach, and the outcomes immediately followed. In David's own words: "Sirtfoods have been a disclosure to my diet. Acquainting

Sirtfoods has permitted me with accomplish a body synthesis and prosperity already inconceivable, making ready for my arrival to the ring and recovering my title as heavyweight boss of the world. I have consistently supported the temperance's of eating plants, and the disclosure of Sirtfoods shows exactly how incredible they are and why we ought to eat a greater amount of them. On the off chance that anybody approaches me my main tip for getting fit as a fiddle, my answer is to begin eating a Sirtfood-rich diet."

KEEPING MUSCLES YOUTHFUL

What's more, it's not simply muscle size. The prolix c impacts of SIRT1 on muscle stretch out to how it works as well. As muscle ages, its capacity to initiate SIRT1 decreases. This makes it less receptive to the advantages of activity and progressively inclined to harm from free radicals and inflammation, which brings about what is known as oxidative pressure. Muscles bit by bit shrink, get more fragile, and weariness all the more without any problem. In any case, in the event that we can expand actuation of SIRT1, we can stop the age-related decay.

To be sure, by initiating SIRT1 to stop the loss of bulk and capacity we ordinarily observe with maturing, we see numerous related medical advantages, including the stopping of bone loss and avoidance of expanded constant foundational inflammation (known as inflammation), just as upgrades in versatility and generally personal satisfaction.

Obviously, at that point, the most recent research shows that the higher the polyphenol substance (and consequently sirtuin-actuating supplements) in the diets of more established individuals, the more noteworthy the insurance they experience against physical execution decrease with age.

Try not to be tricked into deduction these advantages just apply to the old; a long way from it. By the age of twenty-five, the impacts of maturing can start and muscle gradually dissolves, with 10 percent of muscle lost by age forty (despite the fact that general weight will in general increment) and a 40 percent loss by age seventy.

However proof is developing this would all be able to be forestalled and turned around by animating our sirtuin qualities.

Muscle loss, growth, and capacity: sirtuin action assumes a significant job in everything. Stack it up, and it's no big surprise that in an ongoing audit in the lofty clinical diary Nature, sirtuins were depicted as ace controllers of muscle growth, with expanding sirtuin initiation referred to as one of the promising rising roads for fighting muscle loss, and in this manner expanding personal satisfaction just as diminishing infection and passing's.

Seen with regards to the ground-breaking impacts our sirtuin qualities can have on muscles, the stun aftereffects of our pilot preliminary no longer appeared to be so stunning. We started to acknowledge it was conceivable to fuel weight loss while taking care of our muscles, all through a Sirtfood-rich diet.

In any case, that is only the beginning. In the following section we will see the advantages of Sirtfoods broaden such a great amount of further, to all parts of wellbeing and personal satisfaction. **RUNDOWN**

- Despite getting in shape, we discovered, individuals following the Sirtfood Diet either kept up or even picked up muscle. This is on the grounds that sirtuins are ace controllers of muscle.

- By actuating sirtuins, it is conceivable both to forestall muscle breakdown and to advance muscle recovery.

- Activating SIRT1 can likewise assist with forestalling the progressive loss of muscle that we see with maturing.

Not exclusively will actuating your sirtuin qualities make you look more slender, it will assist you with remaining more advantageous and capacity better as you age.

CHAPTER FOUR: WELL-BEING WONDERS IN SIRTFOOD

In spite of all the astounding advances in current medication, society is getting fatter and more wiped out—70 percent of all passing are because of constant malady, a really stunning measurement. Radical change is required, and quick.

However, as we have seen, we can start to change the entirety of this. By actuating our antiquated sirtuin qualities we can consume fat and manufacture a less fatty and more grounded body. Furthermore, with sirtuins at the center point of our digestion, ace software engineers of our science, their significance reaches out a long ways past body organization alone, to each aspect of our prosperity.

SIRTUINS AND THE 70 PERCENT

Think about a sickness that you partner with getting old and the odds are an absence of sirtuin movement in the body is included. For instance, sirtuin initiation is extraordinary for heart wellbeing, ensuring the muscle cells in the heart and by and large helping the heart muscle work better. It likewise improves how our conduits work, causes us handle cholesterol all the more productively, and secures against the stopping up of our supply routes known as atherosclerosis.

What about diabetes? Sirtuin initiation builds the measure of insulin that can be discharged and encourages it work all the more viably in the body. As it occurs, one of the most mainstream subterranean insect diabetic medications, metformin, depends on SIRT1 for its helpful impact. In fact, one pharmaceutical organization is at present exploring adding regular sirtuin activators to metformin treatment for diabetics, with results from creature contemplates indicating an amazing 83 percent decrease in the portion of metformin required for similar impacts.

With regards to the cerebrum, sirtuins are included once more, with sirtuin movement saw as lower in Alzheimer's patients. Conversely, sirtuin enactment improves correspondence flags in the mind, upgrades subjective capacity, and diminishes cerebrum inflammation. This stops the development of amyloid-creation and tau protein conglomeration, two of the primary harming things we see happening in the minds of Alzheimer's patients.

Bones are straightaway. Osteoblasts are an uncommon sort of cell in our bones answerable for building new bone. The more osteoblasts we have, the more grounded our bones.

Sirtuin initiation advances the creation of osteoblast cells, yet in addition expands their endurance. This makes sirtuin initiation fundamental for lifelong bone wellbeing.

Malignant growth has been a progressively questionable region for sirtuin explores, and keeping in mind that ongoing exploration shows that sirtuin initiation assists with smothering disease tumors, researchers are just barely starting to disentangle this complex. While there is considerably more to learn on this specific subject, those societies that eat the most Sirtfoods have the least malignant growth rates, as we will before long observe.

Coronary illness, diabetes, dementia, osteoporosis, and most likely malignant growth: it's an amazing rundown of infections that can be forestalled by enacting sirtuins. It might not shock discover that societies previously eating a lot of Sirtfoods as a major aspect of their customary diets experience a life span and prosperity the majority of us could scarcely envision, which you'll hear more on very soon.

That leaves us with an energizing end: just by including the world's most strong Sirtfoods to your diet, and making that a lifelong propensity, you also can encounter this degree of prosperity—and that's only the tip of the iceberg—all while getting the build you need.

By putting together his nutritional arrangement with respect to Sirtfoods, David can contend at his best, however has totally switched his future danger of coronary illness and diabetes.

CONTEXTUAL INVESTIGATION

David Carr is an expert mariner who is contending in the renowned 2017 America's Cup crusade. David trains like a top competitor, and his diet must be viewed as healthy, including taking enhancements. However in his own words, he was "consistently the fat competitor," and it goaded him that he ate preferred and prepared more earnestly over a significant number of the competitors around him, yet they were less fatty. In spite of all his activity and great diet, he additionally demonstrated hazard factors for metabolic sickness with elevated levels of glucose, cholesterol, and different fats in his blood.

With a Sirtfood-rich diet, including a Sirtfood drink every morning, as the foundation of his nutritional arrangement, David experienced gigantic outcomes. Inside a half year he was down from 229 pounds to his objective weight of 205.

SYNOPSIS

- Despite all the advances in present day medication, as a general public we're getting fatter and more debilitated.
- Seventy percent of all passing are because of incessant malady, with low sirtuin movement involved in by far most.
- By actuating sirtuins, you can forestall or hinder the major interminable infections of the Western world.

By pressing your diet brimming with Sirtfoods, you also can appreciate a similar degree of prosperity as the most advantageous and longest-living populaces on earth.

CHAPTER FIVE: SIRTFOODS

So far we have found that sirtuins are an old group of qualities with the ability to assist us with consuming fat, form muscle, and keep us too healthy. It is settled that sirtuins can be turned on through caloric limitation, fasting, and exercise, yet there is another progressive method to accomplish this: food. We allude to the nourishments generally amazing at actuating sirtuins as Sirtfoods.

PAST CANCER PREVENTION AGENTS

To truly comprehend the advantages of Sirtfoods expects us to contemplate nourishments like foods grown from the ground, and the reasons they are beneficial for us. There's definitely no uncertainty that they are, with heaps of research affirming that diets wealthy in organic products, vegetables, and plant nourishments by and large cut the danger of numerous incessant maladies, including the greatest executioners, coronary illness and malignant growth.

This has been put down to their rich substance of supplements, for example, nutrients, minerals, and, obviously, cancer prevention agents, most likely the greatest wellbeing popular expression of the most recent decade. However, we're here to recount to an altogether different story.

The explanation Sirtfoods are so bravo has nothing to do with those supplements we as a whole know so well and hear such a great amount about. Of course, they are on the whole important things that you have to get from your diet, however there's something out and out various, and exceptionally uncommon, going on with Sirtfoods. Indeed, imagine a scenario where we tossed that entire perspective on its head and said that the explanation Sirtfoods are beneficial for you isn't on the grounds that they sustain the body with basic supplements, or give cancer prevention agents to clean up the harming impacts of free radicals, yet a remarkable inverse: since they are brimming with feeble poisons. In reality as we know it where pretty much every touted "super food" is forcefully showcased based on its cell reinforcement content, this may sound insane. Be that as it may, it's a progressive thought, and one worth understanding.

WHAT DOESN'T EXECUTE YOU MAKES YOU MORE GROUNDED

How about we return to the built up methods of enacting sirtuins for a second: fasting and exercise. As we've seen, explore has more than once indicated that dietary vitality limitation has sensational advantages for weight loss, wellbeing, and conceivably life span. At that point there's activity, with its multitudinous advantages for both body and brain, borne out by the finding that standard exercise drastically slices death rates. Be that as it may, what is the one thing they share for all intents and purpose?

The appropriate response is: stress. Both fasting and exercise cause a mellow weight on the body that urges it to adjust by getting fitter, increasingly effective, and stronger. It's the body's reaction to these somewhat upsetting boosts—its adjustment— that makes us fitter, more beneficial, and more slender over the long haul. Furthermore, as we currently know, these exceptionally gainful adjustments are organized by sirtuins, which are turned on notwithstanding these stressors, and light a large group of ideal changes in the body.

The specialized term for adjustment to these anxieties is hormesis. The thought you get a valuable impact from being presented to a low portion of a substance or stress that is in any case poisonous or deadly whenever given at higher dosages. Or on the other hand, on the off chance that you like, "what doesn't execute you makes you more grounded." And that is actually how fasting and exercise work. Starvation is deadly, and unnecessary exercise is inconvenient to wellbeing. These extraordinary types of pressure are obviously hurtful, however insofar as fasting and exercise stay moderate and reasonable anxieties, they have profoundly gainful impacts.

ENTER POLYPHENOLS

Presently, this is the place things get genuinely intriguing. Every single living creature experience hormesis, however what has been significantly undervalued as of recently is this likewise incorporates plants. While we regularly wouldn't consider plants being equivalent to other living beings, not to mention people, we really share comparable reactions as far as how we respond, on a synthetic level, to our condition.

As amazing as that sounds, it bodes well looking at the situation objectively in transformative terms, since every living thing developed to understanding and adapt to normal ecological anxieties, for example, lack of hydration, daylight, supplement hardship, and assault by pathogens.

Despite that is hard to fold your head over, prepare for the genuinely bewildering bit. Plant pressure reactions are in reality more advanced than our own. Consider it: in the event that we are ravenous and parched, we can go looking for food and drink; excessively hot, we fi conceal; enduring an onslaught, we can escape. In complete differentiation, plants are fixed, and all things considered, they should persevere through all the boundaries of these physiological burdens and dangers. In outcome, in the course of the most recent billion years they have built up an exceptionally modern pressure reaction framework that lowers anything we can gloat. The manner in which they do this is by creating an immense assortment of common plant synthetic compounds—called polyphenols— that permit them to effectively adjust to their condition and endure. At the point when we devour these plants, we additionally expend these polyphenol supplements.

Their impact is significant: they enact our own inborn pressure reaction pathways. We're speaking here about the very same pathways that fasting and exercise switch on: the sirtuins. Piggybacking on a plant's pressure reaction framework along these lines, for our own advantage, is known as xeno- hormesis. Also, the suggestions are down evolving. Let the plants accomplish the difficult work so we don't need to. To be sure, these characteristic plant mixes are presently alluded to as caloric limitation mimetic because of their capacity to turn on similar positive changes in our phones, for example, fat consuming that would be seen during fasting. Also, by furnishing us with further developed flagging mixes than we produce ourselves, they trigger results better than anything we can accomplish through fasting or exercise alone.

Because of a more noteworthy need to adjust to make due in their condition, nourishments developed in the wild or even naturally, are preferable for us over seriously cultivated produce since they produce more significant levels of polyphenols.

SIRTFOODS

While all plants have these pressure reaction frameworks, just certain ones have created to deliver important measures of sirtuin-initiating polyphenols. We call these plants Sirtfoods. Their disclosure implies that rather than somber fasting regimens or difficult exercise programs, there is currently a progressive better approach to actuate your sirtuin qualities: eating a diet inexhaustible in Sirtfoods. The best part is that this one includes putting (Sirt) nourishments onto your plate, not taking them off! It's so wonderfully basic thus simple it appears there must be a trick.

Be that as it may, there isn't. This is the manner by which nature expected us to eat, instead of the stomach thundering or calorie tallying of present day dieting. Huge numbers of you, who have encountered these loathsome diets, where starting weight loss, is temporary before the body rebels and the weight returns heaping on, will justifiably shiver at the idea of another bogus guarantee, another book gloating the feared "d" word. In any case, recollect this: the advanced way to deal with diet is just 150 years of age; Sirtfoods were created ordinarily in excess of a billion years prior.

Also, with that, you're presumably tingling to comprehend what explicit nourishments consider Sirtfoods. So right away, here are the main twenty Sirtfoods.

OUTLINE

- We need to drastically reconsider the possibility that natural products, vegetables, and plant nourishments are beneficial for us essentially on the grounds that they contain nutrients and cancer prevention agents.

- They are beneficial for us since they contain normal synthetic compounds that place a mellow weight on our cells, similarly as fasting and exercise do.

- Plants, in light of the fact that they are fixed, have built up an exceptionally advanced pressure reaction framework and produce polyphenols to assist them with adjusting to the difficulties of their condition.

- When we eat these plants, their polyphenols initiate our pressure reaction pathways—our sirtuin qualities—mirroring the impacts of caloric limitation and exercise.

The nourishments with the most remarkable sirtuin-enacting impacts are called Sirtfoods.

CHAPTER SIX: SIRTFOODS AROUND THE GLOBE

Sirtfoods might be an ongoing nutritional revelation, yet plainly various societies have been encountering their advantages since the beginning. As we become increasingly acquainted with the main twenty Sirtfoods in part 8, we will perceive what number of have been venerated since early development for their therapeutic properties and were frequently viewed as hallowed nourishments for their capacity to present power and prosperity.

Truth be told, it currently gives the idea that put down accounts of such advantages of Sirtfoods go route back to being the subject of the very rest clinical preliminary at any point recorded. Reported over 2,200 years back, we discover it in the Book of Daniel in the Good book. What was seen to be the best accessible food of the day was endorsed to keep the youngsters healthy and t so they could later enter the ruler's administration.

However apparently, when this was tested by Daniel, a diet of just plants delivered a predominant result in simply a question of days: "Daniel decided not to let himself become customarily unclean by eating the rich food and drinking the wine of the regal court. . . . So Daniel went to the watchman . . . Test us for ten days, he said. Give us vegetables [plants] to eat and water to drink. At that point contrast us and the youngsters who are eating the food of the illustrious court, and base your choice on what we look like. He consented to let them attempt it for ten days.

At the point when the time was up, it was seen that they were better in appearance and fatter in tissue [muscular] than every one of the individuals who had been eating the illustrious food. So from that point on the gatekeeper let them keep on eating vegetables rather than what the ruler gave." Such advantages, particularly expanded bulk, could never regularly be normal from a diet of just plants. That is, obviously, except if those plants happened to be amazingly rich Sirtfood sources.

With records indicating that the regular plants expended in those days were like the Sirtfood-rich conventional Mediterranean diet, and the outcomes strikingly like our own pilot preliminary, one can't yet ponder whether the Daniel preliminary is the stuff of tale, or have we accidentally had the response to accomplishing the body and wellbeing we've generally wanted for over two centuries?

ENTER THE BLUE ZONE

While our wellbeing is weak, there are locales around the globe, named Blue Zones, where the admission of Sirtfoods is a whole lot higher than the sum we expend in a common Western diet. Undoubtedly, for the way of life eating Sirtfood rich diets, the advantages appear to be progressively similar to the stuff of legend.

Truth be told, in addition to the fact that we see individuals living longer in Blue Zones than in nations where a run of the mill Western diet is the standard, however substantially more significant is the manner by which they hold young essentialness in mature age. In the Blue Zones, there are unbelievably low paces of Alzheimer's, malignant growth, diabetes, coronary illness, and osteoporosis. Go there and you will see individuals matured ninety or more established strolling, moving, and working. They are not dynamic in the interest to get in shape; there's no need—there are no rec centers. Rather they hold the life and vitality of youth into mature age. You will see them on bikes or riding bikes in the road.

Get visiting to them and you may hear them brag about how extraordinary their sexual coexistence despite everything is! What's more, it is nothing unexpected that they additionally happen to be the slimmest populaces on the planet.

I SHOULD COCOA

To all the more likely comprehend this mind boggling wonder, how about we start our excursion with an outing to the San Blas

Islands of Panama, the indigenous home of the Kuna Native Americans, who seem resistant to hypertension and show amazingly low paces of corpulence, diabetes, malignant growth, and early passing. At the turn of the twenty-first century, an exploration group uncovered the Kuna's mystery when they found that their significant wellspring of liquid was a drink produced using privately developed cocoa. This cocoa is fabulously wealthy in a particular gathering of polyphenols called avanols, particularly epicatechin, which qualifies it as a Sirtfood.

Be that as it may, how might we realize that the hearty wellbeing of the Kuna was owing to their high admission of cocoa avanols? The scientists found that when the Kuna Indians moved to Panama

City and changed to expending seriously prepared business cocoa (which is deprived of its avanols and in this way not, at this point a Sirtfood), the medical advantages evaporated.

The instance of the Kuna is nevertheless one piece in a developing collection of proof that avanol- rich cocoa has phenomenal medical advantages. In clinical investigations, avanol-rich cocoa has been found to improve circulatory strain, blood stream, glucose control, and cholesterol measures. Audits recommend that cocoa likewise has constructive outcomes in diabetes4 and malignant growth.

Utilization has been appeared to upgrade memory execution, proffering an important dietary choice in the quest for the cerebrum's wellspring of youth. What's more, in spite of the oft-rehashed admonitions that chocolate is awful for you, we currently realize that cocoa improves oral cleanliness and shields teeth from plaque and cavities.

ZEST FOREVER

Turmeric, known as "Indian strong gold," has been utilized in Ayurveda medication for over 4,000 years for its injury mending and hostile to inflammatory properties. We currently realize these recuperating impacts are because of the way that it contains curcumin, a significant sirtuin-enacting supplement, which makes it a Sirtfood.

Turmeric is a predominant zest in conventional Indian cooking and is accepted to add to the way that malignancy rates in India are essentially lower than in Western nations. However strikingly, the disease rate for Indians increments by 50 to 75 percent when they move from India to the US or UK and relinquish their customary diet.8 While this may be because of various distinctive lifestyle factors, logical proof currently shows that curcumin has powerful anticancer properties.

Notwithstanding its anticancer cases, there is mounting proof of other sirtuin-enacting medical advantages. In late examinations, an uncommon type of curcumin that was made to be all the more handily consumed was appeared to improve cholesterol levels, improve glucose control, and diminish inflammation in the body. It has been explored for osteoarthritis of the knee and demonstrated to be as powerful as ordinarily taken painkillers. Analysts are presently revealing its numerous systems for forestalling weight addition and assisting with treating obesity. And in patients with early sort 2 diabetes, simply eating a gram of turmeric daily improved their working memory.

GREEN LIVING

Green tea is another enticing Sirtfood offering. Green tea utilization is thought to have started over 4,700 years prior when the Chinese head ("Divine Healer") created a charming, reviving drink with green tea leaves by good fortune. It was just a lot later that the drink built up its notoriety for restorative and mending ability.

Asia's high admission of green tea has been referred to as a key purpose behind the "Asian Catch 22." Notwithstanding a very high commonness of cigarette smoking, Asia, and particularly Japan, brags some the most reduced paces of cardiovascular infection and lung malignancy on the planet. A high admission of green tea is connected with much lower paces of coronary illness and a diminished danger of numerous regular diseases, for example, those influencing the prostate, stomach, lung, and bosom. It is little miracle in this manner that green tea utilization is connected to significantly less early passing..

Green tea additionally has a thermo genic impact, which implies it builds the measure of vitality the body consumes off, helping fat loss while looking after muscle. Consolidate green tea with a diet plenteous in verdant greens, soy, herbs, and flavors (turmeric use is particularly common), to make a buffet of Sirtfoods, and we have a diet fundamentally the same as that found in Okinawa—"the place where there is the immortals." Okinawa may be the least fortunate territory in Japan, yet it holds the record for life span and the best number of centenarians on the planet.

So bewildering is their personal satisfaction, scientists accepted it must be a direct result of prevalent qualities. Be that as it may, along came the Westernization of its diet, and with it blossoming paces of weight and devastating infections that more youthful ages are currently encountering just because, immovably settling any thought of prevalent qualities.

A MEDITERRANEAN SOLUTION

For a genuine abundance of Sirtfood blends, we have to venture out to the Mediterranean. This is the place we locate the meeting up of a large group of intense Sirtfoods, in particular additional virgin olive oil, nuts, berries, green verdant vegetables, herbs and flavors, and, obviously, wine.

Eating this kind of diet is connected to a 9 percent decrease in death from all causes, with generous decreases in cardiovascular infection and degenerative mind sicknesses like Alzheimer's, just as malignancy.

What's more, as we found in our presentation, the milestone PREDIMED preliminary, did in Spain, found that a Mediterranean-style diet enhanced with either additional virgin olive oil or nuts (particularly pecans) cut the frequency of cardiovascular ailment and diabetes.

Analysts additionally accomplished something intriguing in a sub investigation of PREDIMED. They analyzed the hereditary expert le for PPAR-γ—which, on the off chance that you recall, is the stoutness reprobate we ran over before. While a few of us are very impervious to its activities, others are not all that lucky, and can truly get clobbered by it. This implies you may eat equivalent to another person yet be significantly more powerless to weight gain. In any case, it shouldn't be that path with Sirtfoods.

In the individuals who followed the Sirtfood-rich Mediterranean diet, the negative impacts of this quality were turned around. Unbelievably, in spite of no drop in calories, the diet more extravagant in Sirtfoods was connected to a 40 percent drop in the danger of heftiness, particularly weight put away around the belly. Disregard low fat and overlook fixating on calories: the individuals who follow a conventional Mediterranean diet will consistently be slimmer than everybody.

So there we have it.

The way of life around the globe whose individuals are most advantageous and slimmest and live the longest lives share something practically speaking: they eat the most elevated measure of Sirtfoods. They remain lean and thin without to such an extent as checking a calorie or starting a better eating routine. That leaves us to do only a certain something, which is to sort out the entirety of the most intense Sirtfoods on earth to make a diet any semblance of which has never been seen— fundamentally, a diet to drive a wellbeing and weight-loss insurgency.

RUNDOWN

- While weight and incessant sickness are wild in the Western world, there are Blue Zones that are for all intents and purposes insusceptible to these issues.

- One thing that individuals living in Blue Zones share for all intents and purpose is a diet rich in Sirtfoods.

- Classic models incorporate the Kuna Native Americans with their propensity for cocoa, the turmeric-implanted diet of India, the Japanese preference for green tea, and the additional virgin olive oil at the core of the customary Mediterranean diet.

  The Sirtfood Diet unites all these incredible nourishments—and that's only the tip of the iceberg— into a world-beating diet for wellbeing and weight loss.

CHAPTER SEVEN: BUILDING A DIET THAT WORKS FOR YOU

With the Sirtfood Diet, we have accomplished something extraordinary. We've taken the most intense Sirtfoods on earth and have woven them into a fresh out of the box better approach for eating, any semblance of which has never been seen. We have chosen the "most elite" from the most advantageous diets at any point known and from them made a world-beating diet.

The uplifting news is, you don't need to abruptly receive the customary diet of an Okinawan or have the option to cook like an Italian mamma. That is totally ridiculous, yet absolutely superfluous on the Sirtfood Diet. In reality, one thing that may strike you from the rundown of Sirtfoods is their commonality. While you may not presently be eating all the nourishments on the rundown, you in all probability are devouring a few. So for what reason would you say you are not previously getting thinner?

The appropriate response is discovered when we analyze the various components that the most bleeding edge nutritional science shows are required for building a diet that works. It's tied in with eating Sirtfoods in the correct amount, assortment, and structure. It's tied in with supplementing Sirtfood dishes with liberal servings of protein, and afterward eating your dinners at the best time of day. What's more, it's about the opportunity to eat the truly delicious nourishments that you appreciate in the sums you like.

HITTING YOUR SHARE

At the present time, a great many people essentially don't devour about enough Sirtfoods to evoke a powerful fat-consuming and wellbeing boosting impact. At the point when analysts took a gander at utilization of five key sirtuin-enacting supplements in the US diet, they saw singular day by day admissions as a tightfisted 13 milligrams for every day.1 interestingly, the normal Japanese admission was multiple times higher.2 Contrast that and our Sirtfood Diet preliminary, where people were expending several milligrams of sirtuin-actuating supplements each day.

What we are discussing is an all-out diet transformation where we increment our everyday admission of sirtuin-actuating supplements by as much as ftyfold. While this may sound overwhelming or unfeasible, it truly isn't. By taking all our top Sirtfoods and assembling them in a manner that is absolutely perfect with your bustling life, you also can without much of a stretch and viably arrive at the degree of admission expected to receive all the rewards.

THE INTENSITY OF COOPERATIVE ENERGY

We trust it is smarter to devour a wide scope of these marvel supplements as common entire nourishments, where they exist together close by the many other regular bioactive plant synthetic concoctions that demonstration synergistically to help our wellbeing. We think it is smarter to work with nature, as opposed to against it. It's consequently that over and over enhancements of secluded supplements neglect to show enduring advantage, yet exactly the same supplement when given all in all food does.

Take, for instance, the exemplary sirtuin-enacting supplement resveratrol. In supplement structure, it is ineffectively ingested; yet in its characteristic food lattice of red wine, its bioavailability (how much the body can utilize) is in any event multiple times higher. Add to this the way that red wine contains one as well in general scope of sirtuin-enacting polyphenols that demonstration together to bring medical advantages, including piceatannol, quercetin, myricetin, and epicatechin.

Or on the other hand we may change our consideration regarding curcumin from turmeric. Curcumin is entrenched to be the key sirtuin-initiating supplement in turmeric, yet look into shows that entire turmeric has better PPAR-γ action for battling fat loss and is increasingly powerful at repressing malignant growth and lessening glucose levels than curcumin in isolation.5 It's not hard to perceive any reason why disconnecting a solitary supplement is not even close as compelling as expending it in its entire food structure.

In any case, what makes a dietary methodology extremely uncommon is the point at which we start to consolidate various Sirtfoods. For instance, by including quercetin-rich Sirtfoods, we improve the bioavailability of resveratrol-containing nourishments significantly further. This, yet their activities supplement one another. Both are fat busters, yet there are subtleties in how every one of them accomplishes this.

Resveratrol is viable at assisting with crushing existing fat cells, while quercetin exceeds expectations in forestalling new fat cell formation.6 in blend they target fat from the two sides, bringing about a more noteworthy effect on fat loss than if we just ate a lot of a solitary food.

What's more, this is an example we see again and again. Nourishments rich in the sirtuin activator apigenin improve the assimilation of quercetin from food, and upgrade its activity. Thus, quercetin has been appeared to synergize with the movement of epigallocatechin gallate (EGCG). And EGCG has been appeared to work synergistically with curcumin.9 Thus it goes on. In addition to the fact that individual are entire nourishments more strong than secluded supplements, yet by joining Sirtfoods we tap into an entire embroidery of medical advantages that nature has weaved—so many-sided, so re fined, it is difficult to attempt to best it.

SQUEEZING AND FOOD: OUTDO THE TWO UNIVERSES

The two juices and entire nourishments are indispensable to the Sirtfood Diet. Here, we are discussing juices explicitly made utilizing a juicer—blenders and smoothie producers, (for example, the NutriBullet) won't work. For some, this will appear to be strange, on the premise that when something is squeezed the fiber is expelled. Be that as it may, for verdant greens this is actually what we need.

The fiber from food contains what are called non-extractable polyphenols (or NEPPs). These are polyphenols, including sirtuin activators that are joined to the sinewy piece of the food and are possibly discharged when separated by our neighborly gut microscopic organisms. By evacuating the fiber, we don't get the NEPPs and miss out on their decency. However, significantly, the NEPP content differs drastically relying upon the sort of plant.

The NEPP substance of nourishments like natural product, oats, and nuts is huge, and these ought to be eaten entire (in strawberries, NEPPs give in excess of 50 percent of the polyphenols!). Be that as it may, for verdant vegetables, the dynamic fixings in the Sirtfood juice, they are far lower regardless of a huge majority of fiber.

So with regards to verdant greens, we get most extreme value for our money by squeezing them and evacuating the low-supplement fiber, which means we can utilize a lot more prominent volumes and accomplish an excessively thought hit of sirtuin-actuating polyphenols.

There is additionally another favorable position to expelling the fiber. Verdant greens contain a sort of fiber called insoluble fiber, which has a scouring activity in the stomach related framework. In any case, when we eat a lot of it, much the same as on the off chance that we over scour something, it can bother and harm our gut lining. That implies verdant green–stuffed smoothies will be fiber over- burden for some individuals, conceivably exasperating or in any event, causing IBS (bad tempered gut disorder) and preventing our assimilation of supplements.

Having a portion of your Sirtfoods in juice structure can likewise have huge favorable circumstances with regards to engrossing their integrity. For instance, one of the fixings we remember for the green juice is coordinate a green tea. At the point when we devour the sirtuin activator EGCG, found in significant levels in green tea, in drink structure without food, its assimilation is in excess of 65 percent higher. We additionally think that it's intriguing to take note of that when we ran blood tests on our own customers, changing from smoothies to green juices achieved emotional increments in their degrees of other basic supplements, for example, magnesium and folic corrosive.

The core, all things considered, is that to truly get those sirtuin qualities ring for emotional weight loss and wellbeing, we have to manufacture a diet that joins the two juices and entire nourishments for most extreme advantage.

THE INTENSITY OF PROTEIN

Its plants that put the Sirt into the Sirtfood Diet, however to receive most extreme reward, Sirtfood suppers ought to consistently be wealthy in protein. A structure square of dietary protein called leucine has been appeared to have extra advantages in animating SIRT1 to expand fat consuming and improve glucose control.

Be that as it may, leucine additionally has another job, and this is the place its synergistic relationship with Sirtfoods truly sparkles. Leucine powerfully animates anabolism (building things) in our phones, especially in muscle, which requests a great deal of vitality and means our vitality production lines (called mitochondria) need to stay at work past 40 hours. This makes a need in our cells for the movement of Sirtfoods. As you may review, one of the impacts of Sirtfoods is to animate more mitochondria to be made, improve how effective they are, and make them consume fat as fuel. Consequently our bodies need them to satisfy this additional vitality need.

The end result is that by joining Sirtfoods with dietary protein, we see a synergistic impact that supports sirtuin initiation and at last make you consume fat to fuel muscle growth and better wellbeing. This is the reason the dinners in the book are intended to give a liberal serving of protein. Sleek fish are an astoundingly decent protein decision to supplement the activity of Sirtfoods, as they are wealthy in omega-3 unsaturated fats notwithstanding their protein content. You will without a doubt have heard parts about the medical advantages of sleek fish and explicitly omega-3 fish oils. Furthermore, presently late research is proposing that the advantages of omega-3 fats may come through improving how our sirtuin qualities work.

There have been concerns raised about the negative impacts of protein-rich diets on wellbeing as of late, and without Sirtfoods to offset the protein, we can start to get why. Leucine can be a twofold edged blade. As we've seen, we need Sirtfoods to enable our cells to fulfill the metabolic need that leucine puts on them. Yet, without them, our mitochondria can get broken, and as opposed to improving wellbeing, high leucine levels can really advance stoutness and insulin opposition.

Sirtfoods help to keep the impacts of leucine within proper limits as well as effectively working in our flavor. Consider leucine squeezing your foot on the quickening agent of weight loss and prosperity, with Sirtfoods the apparatus that guarantees the cell fulfills the expanded need. Without the Sirtfoods, the motor blows. . . .

Returning to worries about the wellbeing impacts of protein-rich diets, Sirtfoods are the missing bit of the riddle. The US diet is ordinarily protein rich, however missing Sirtfoods to offset it. This makes it imperative that Sirtfoods become a fundamental piece of how Americans eat.

EAT EARLY

With regards to eating, our way of thinking is the previous the better, in a perfect world completing the process of eating for the day by 7 p.m. This is for two reasons. To begin with, to procure the characteristic satisfying impact of Sirtfoods. There's significantly more advantage to eating a supper that will keep you feeling full, fulfilled, and stimulated as you approach your day than spending the entire day feeling hungry just to eat and remain full as you stay asleep from sundown to sunset.

However, there is a second convincing explanation, which is to continue dietary patterns in line with your interior body clock. We as a whole have a worked in body clock, considered our circadian cadence that directs a significant number of our normal body capacities as indicated by the hour of day. In addition to other things, it impacts how the body handles the food we eat. Our checks work in synchrony, essentially following the signs of the light-dim pattern of the sun. As diurnal animal groups, we're intended to be dynamic in the daytime instead of around evening time. Therefore, our body clock gears us up to deal with food most effectively during the day, when it is light and we are relied upon to be dynamic, and less so when it is dull, where we are rather prepared for rest and rest.

The issue is that a large number of us have "work tickers" and "social timekeepers" that are not in a state of harmony with the shutting down of the sun. After dull is here and there the main possibility a few of us get the opportunity to eat. To a certain extent, we can prepare our body clock to synchronize to various timetables, for example, "evening chronotypes" who like or must be dynamic, eat, and rest later in the day. Be that as it may, living skewed from the outside light-dull cycle includes some significant pitfalls. This is actually what we see among night-move laborers, who have higher paces of corpulence and metabolic ailment, which is in any event mostly because of the impacts of their late eating designs.

The consequence is that you're in an ideal situation eating prior in the day whenever the situation allows, preferably by 7 p.m. In any case, consider the possibility that this is simply not doable.

Fortunately sirtuins assume a key job in body clock synchronization. Truth be told, investigate has discovered that the polyphenols in Sirtfoods are fit for tweaking our body tickers and emphatically modifying circadian rhythm that implies on the off chance that you basically can't abstain from eating later, the incorporation of Sirtfoods with your feast will limit the impeding impacts. Without a doubt, one of the repetitive bits of input we get notification from supporters of the Sirtfood Diet is exactly how much their rest quality has improved, proposing intense impacts on blending their circadian beat.

PULL OUT ALL THE STOPS ON TASTE

A major issue with customary dieting is that it normally makes for a hopeless feasting experience. It depletes each and every drop of delight from food, leaving us feeling disappointed. In any case, for us, it's fundamental that you keep up the delight of food in the quest for a healthy weight. That is the reason we were pleased when we understood that Sirtfoods, just as the nourishments that improve their activity, for example, protein and omega-3 food sources, are prepared to fulfill our craving for taste. It's a definitive success win: the Sirtfood Diet supports our wellbeing and tastes incredible.

How about we return a stage to perceive how this functions. Our taste buds decide how scrumptious we discover our food, and how fulfilled we are from eating it. This is done through seven significant taste receptors. Over innumerable ages, people have advanced to search out the preferences that animate these receptors so as to accomplish greatest sustenance from our diet. The better a food animates these taste receptors, the more fulfillments we get from a feast.

Also, in the Sirtfood Diet we have a definitive menu for upbeat taste buds, since it offers most extreme incitement over all taste receptors. To sum up these preferences and the nourishments you'll eat on the diet that fulfill them: the seven significant taste sensations are sweet (strawberries, dates); salty (celery, fish); harsh (strawberries); unpleasant (cocoa, kale, endive, additional virgin olive oil, green tea); sharp (chilies, garlic, additional virgin olive oil); astringent (green tea, red wine); and umami (soy, fish, meat).

Urgently, what we have found is that the more prominent the sirtuin-actuating properties of a food, the more intensely it animates those taste communities, and the more satisfaction we get from the food we eat. Significantly, it additionally implies that we fulfill our craving faster, and our longing to eat more is decreased in like manner. This is a key motivation behind why the individuals who follow a Sirtfood-rich diet are enjoyably fuller more rapidly.

For instance, normal cocoa has a striking, engaging severe taste, however expel the sirtuin-enacting avanols with forceful mechanical food preparing procedures and we are left with mass-created, dull, and characterless cocoa that is utilized to make profoundly sugared chocolate confectionary. By this point, the medical advantages have disappeared.

A similar standard applies to olive oil. Devoured in its negligibly prepared structure—additional virgin—it has a ground-breaking and particular flavor, with a strengthening kick that can be felt at the rear of the throat. However re fined and handled olive oil loses all character, is mellow and dull, and conveys no such kick. So also, hot chilies gloat a lot more noteworthy sirtuin-enacting accreditations than the milder assortments, and wild strawberries are a lot more delectable than cultivated ones because of a more extravagant substance of sirtuin-actuating supplements.

Not just this, we likewise locate that individual Sirtfoods can trigger various taste receptors: green tea is both unpleasant and astringent, and strawberries have a blend of prepared flavors.

At first, a few palates won't be acclimated with sure of these flavors—such an extensive amount our cutting edge food is without the two supplements and genuine taste—yet you will be flabbergasted how rapidly you obtain an adoration for them. All things considered, people developed to search out a diet rich in Sirtfoods, close by restorative protein and omega-3 unsaturated fats, to fulfill the fundamental wants of our hunger and, thusly, our wellbeing. This developmental procedure happened over centuries, without us knowing the reasons, yet it guaranteed we got greatest profit by devouring these nourishments.

GRASP EATING

How about we attempt a test. We simply need you to do one extremely straightforward thing for us: don't think about a white bear.

What did you simply consider? A white bear, obviously. Why? Since we instructed you not to. Try not to reveal to us you are as yet pondering it!

This was the trailblazing test performed by brain research teacher Daniel Wegner in 1987, which demonstrated that constrained concealment of considerations causes a dumbfounding and counterproductive heightening in how regularly we really consider what we are attempting to suppress. So as opposed to blocking it from our contemplations, the exertion delivers a distraction with the stifled idea.

Furthermore, as you've presumably speculated, this marvel isn't relevant just to white bears. Precisely the same thing happens when we make antagonists of and confine nourishments for weight loss. Studies show we really consider them all the more frequently, expanding allurement. It consumes us until we eat it! Also, with the diet broken and the heightened pondering the "prohibited" nourishments we suffered, we are presently significantly more prone to gorge.

Researchers have now clarified what's going on here. We as a whole have a profound should be self- governing. At the point when we feel controlled, for example, going on a severe diet, it makes a negative situation that causes us to feel uncomfortable. We feel hostages of this cynicism and revolutionary to break out of it. We rebel by doing what we were told we ought not, and doing it much more than we would have in any case. It happens to us all, even the most self-controlled. It is anything but a matter of if, however when. Researchers presently accept this is a basic motivation behind why we can keep up diets and even get brings about the underlying stages yet neglect to see long haul achievement.

So does this mean there is no reason for endeavoring to change our dietary patterns? Is it accurate to say that we are simply bound for disappointment? No, it implies that when we roll out an improvement, so as to succeed we have to make it our own positive, wanted choice. We presently realize the best approach to accomplish this isn't through dietary rejection yet through dietary consideration. As opposed to concentrating your vitality on the negatives of what try not to eat, rather you center on the positives of what you ought to eat. By doing this, you maintain a strategic distance from the mental backfire. What's more, this is the excellence of the Sirtfood Diet. It's about what you put into your diet, not what you take out. It's about the nature of your food, not the amount. What's more, it's about you needing to do it since you feel fulfilled by eating extraordinary tasting nourishments with the additional information that each nibble gives an abundance of advantages.

Most diets are a necessary chore. They're tied in with holding tight, attempting to keep sight of the "slender perfect." At the end of the day that seldom precedes the diet fizzles, and regardless of whether it is accomplished, it's once in a while continued. The Sirtfood Diet is extraordinary. It is about the excursion. Stage 1, which restricts calories, is kept deliberately quick and painless to guarantee it is done with propelling outcomes before any negative kickback. At that point the emphasis is exclusively on Sirtfoods.

What's more, the inspiration for eating Sirtfoods is driven not simply by a final product of weight loss. Rather it is so a lot if not increasingly about the gratefulness and pleasure in genuine nourishment for a healthy and t lifestyle.

OUTLINE

- The Sirtfood Diet takes the strongest Sirtfoods on earth and unites them in a basic and handy method of eating.

- To accomplish ideal outcomes for weight loss and wellbeing, it is important to eat Sirtfoods in the correct amount, blend, and structures to receive the synergistic rewards of their sirtuin-enacting mixes.

- We further upgrade this by including other healthy fixings, for example, leucine-rich protein nourishments and sleek fish, to make the impacts of the Sirtfood Diet significantly progressively ground-breaking.

- When we eat is likewise significant, and eating prior in the day assists with keeping us on top of our implicit body clock.

- Unlike our advanced diets, Sirtfoods fulfill all our taste receptors, which implies we get more satisfaction from our food and feel content all the more rapidly.

  The Sirtfood Diet is a diet of consideration—not prohibitions, making it the main kind of diet that can convey long haul weight-loss achievement.

CHAPTER EIGHT: TOP TWENTY SIRTFOODS DIET

Since you thoroughly understand Sirtfoods, why they are so incredible and the stuff to make a successful diet that conveys enduring results, it's a great opportunity to begin. In the following section, the very beginning of the Sirtfood Diet starts. So this is simply the ideal time to acclimate with every one of the best twenty Sirtfoods that will before long become staples of your regular diet. **ARUGULA**

Arugula (otherwise called rocket) surely has a beautiful history in US food culture. An impactful green serving of mixed greens leaf with an unmistakable peppery taste, it immediately climbed from humble roots as the base of numerous worker dishes in the Mediterranean to turn into an image of food snootiness in the US, in any event, prompting the instituting of the term arugulance (the meeting up of arugula with egotism)!

Be that as it may, sometime before it was a plate of mixed greens leaf employed in a class war, arugula was respected by the old Greeks and Romans for its therapeutic properties. Regularly utilized as a diuretic and stomach related guide, it picked up its actual popularity from its notoriety for having powerful Spanish fly properties, to such an extent that growth of arugula was restricted in religious communities in the Medieval times, and the well-known Roman artist Virgil composed that "the rocket energizes the sexual want of sleepy individuals." What de nitely energizes us about arugula; however, are its guard levels of the sirtuin-enacting supplements kaempferol and quercetin. Notwithstanding amazing sirtuin-actuating properties, a mix of kaempferol and quercetin is being explored as a restorative fixing in light of the fact that together they saturate and upgrade collagen union in the skin. With those certifications, it's a great opportunity to drop any elitist tag and settle on this the leaf of decision for serving of mixed greens bases, where it matches impeccably with an additional virgin olive oil dressing, joining to make an intense Sirtfood twofold act.

BUCKWHEAT

Buckwheat was perhaps the most punctual harvest to be tamed in Japan, and the story goes that when Buddhist priests made long excursions into the mountains, all they would bring was a cooking pot and a sack of buckwheat for food. So nutritious is buckwheat this was all they required, and it fed them for a considerable length of time. We are enormous buckwheat fans as well. Right off the bat, since it is a standout amongst other known wellsprings of a sirtuin activator called rutin. Yet in addition since it has benefits as a spread harvest, improving soil quality and smothering weed growth, making it an incredible yield for biological and feasible cultivating

One explanation that buckwheat is head and shoulders above other progressively regular grains is presumably that it's anything but a grain by any stretch of the imagination—it's really an organic product seed identified with rhubarb. It would be progressively well-suited to allude to it as a "pseudo-grain." Having one of the most noteworthy protein substances of any grain, just as being a Sirtfood powerhouse, makes it an unmatched option in contrast to all the more ordinarily utilized grains. Also, it is as flexible as any grain proceeding to be, normally without gluten, is an extraordinary decision for the individuals who are gluten prejudiced.

TRICKS

In the event that you're not all that acquainted with escapades, we're discussing those salty, dull green, pellet like things that you may have just had event to see on a pizza. However they are without a doubt one of the most underestimated and neglected nourishments out there.

Intriguingly, they're really the bloom buds of the trick hedge, which develops copiously in the Mediterranean, before being handpicked and saved. Studies presently uncover that escapades have significant antimicrobial, insect diabetic, hostile to inflammatory, safe modulatory and antiviral properties, and they have a rich history of being utilized as a medication in the Mediterranean and North Africa. Scarcely astounding when we find that they are packed loaded with sirtuin-enacting supplements

We believe it's about time these minuscule pieces, so regularly dominated by the other substantial hitters from the Mediterranean diet, and had a lot of greatness. Flavor-wise it's an instance of enormous things coming in little bundles, as they sure sneak up all of a sudden. Be that as it may, in case you're curious about utilizing them, don't feel threatened. We'll before long have you up to speed and falling head over heels for these small supplement hotshots, which when joined with the correct fixings give a wonderfully unmistakable and supreme sharp/salty flavor to adjust a dish in style.

CELERY

Celery has been near and venerated for centuries—with leaves discovered enhancing the remaining parts of the Egyptian pharaoh, who passed on around 1323 BCE. Early strains were unpleasant, and celery was typically viewed as a therapeutic plant particularly for purging and detoxing to forestall disease. That is especially intriguing considering the way that liver, kidney, and gut wellbeing are among the large number of promising advantages that science is currently illustrating.

It was trained as a vegetable in the seventeenth century, and particular reproducing lessened its solid harsh flavor in kind of better assortments, in this way building up its place as a conventional serving of mixed greens vegetable.

With regards to celery, it is critical to take note of that there are two sorts: whitened/yellow and Pascal/green. Whitening is a method that was created to diminish celery's trademark harsh taste, which was seen to be excessively solid. This includes concealing the celery from daylight preceding reaping, bringing about a paler shading and milder flavor. What a tragedy that is, for just as stupefying the flavor, whitening impairs celery's sirtuin-initiating properties. Fortunately the tide is changing and individuals are requesting genuine and unmistakable flavor and are turning around to the more clear green assortment. Green celery is the sort we suggest that you use in both the green juices and dinners, with the most nutritious parts being the hearts and the leaves.

CHILIES

For a large number of years, the stew has been a vital piece of gastronomic experience far and wide. On one level, it is puzzling that we would be so fascinated of it. Its sharp warmth, activated by a substance in chilies called capsaicin, is structured as a plant barrier instrument to cause torment and prevent predators from devouring it, yet we relish it. There is something practically enchanted about the food and our captivation by it. Extraordinarily, one investigation indicated that eating chilies together even expands participation between people. What's more, from a wellbeing viewpoint, we realize that their enchanting warmth is incredible for initiating our sirtuins and boosting our digestion. The bean stew's culinary applications are unending as well, making it a simple method to give any dish a weighty Sirtfood support.

While we value that not every person is an enthusiast of hot or hot food, we trust we can lure you to consider including chilies in limited quantities, particularly considering ongoing examination demonstrating that the individuals who eat fiery nourishments at least three times each week have a 14 percent lower passing rate contrasted with the individuals who eat them not exactly once per week.

When in doubt, the sultrier the stew, the better its Sirtfood qualifications, yet is reasonable and sticks with what is fit to your own preferences. Serrano peppers are an incredible beginning—while at the same time pressing warmth, they are mediocre for a great many people; and for increasingly experienced warmth searchers, we suggest searching out Thai chilies for most extreme sirtuin- enacting benefits. These can be progressively hard to track down in supermarkets however can frequently be found in Asian forte markets. Pick peppers with profound hues, maintaining a strategic distance from those that look wrinkled and delicate.

COCOA

We saw the great medical advantages of cocoa on pages 59–60, so it's nothing unexpected to discover that for antiquated developments, for example, the Aztecs and Mayans, cocoa was viewed as a consecrated food and normally saved for the first class and the warriors, being served at dining experiences to pick up dedication and commitment. Undoubtedly, the cocoa bean was held in such high respect that it was even utilized as a type of cash. In those days it was typically filled in as a foamy beverage. Be that as it may, what could be a progressively flavorful method of getting our dietary cocoa amount than through chocolate? Tsk-tsk, the weakened, refined, and exceptionally improved milk chocolate we ordinarily crunch doesn't tally here. To gain its Sirtfood identification, we are discussing chocolate with 85 percent cocoa solids. Be that as it may, and, after it's all said and done, cocoa rate aside, not all chocolate is made equivalent. Chocolate is regularly treated with an alkalizing specialist (known as Dutch procedure) to lessen its causticity and give it a darker shading. Unfortunately, this procedure enormously decreases its sirtuin initiating avanols, along these lines truly trading off its wellbeing advancing characteristics.

Luckily, and not at all like in numerous different nations, food marking guidelines in the US require that alkalized cocoa must be pronounced all things considered and named "handled with antacid." We suggest maintaining a strategic distance from these items, regardless of whether they gloat a higher cocoa rate, and rather selecting those that have not experienced Dutch preparing to receive the genuine rewards of cocoa.

COFFEE

What's this about coffee as a Sirtfood? We hear you state. We can guarantee you it is anything but a grammatical mistake. Gone are the days when our delight in espresso should have been tempered by a twinge of blame. The examination is unequivocal: espresso is a bona de wellbeing food. Truth be told, it is an authentic fortune trove of fabulous sirtuin actuating supplements. Also, with the greater part of Americans drinking espresso consistently (as much as $40 billion every year!), espresso brags the honor being the main wellspring of polyphenols in the American diet. A definitive incongruity being that the one thing that such huge numbers of wellbeing "specialists" chastised us for doing was really the best thing we were doing every day for our wellbeing. This is the reason espresso consumers have essentially less diabetes, just as lower paces of certain cancers4 and neurodegenerative ailment.

Concerning that extreme incongruity, rather than being a poison, espresso really ensures our livers and makes them healthier!6 And as opposed to the prevalent view that espresso gets dried out the body, it is currently entrenched not to be the situation, with espresso (and furthermore tea) contributing entirely well to the liquid admission of routine espresso consumers. So while we welcome that espresso isn't for everybody, and a few people can be touchy with the impacts of caffeine, for the individuals who appreciate a cup of Joe, its cheerful days.

ADDITIONAL VIRGIN OLIVE OIL

Olive oil is the most eminent food of the conventional Mediterranean diet. The olive tree, otherwise called the "undying tree," is among the most established known developed trees on the planet. Also, its oil has been venerated since the time individuals began to crush olives in stone mortars to gather it, right around 7,000 years prior. Hippocrates referred to it as a fix every one of the; two or after three centuries, present day science currently unequivocally asserts its great medical advantages.

There is presently an abundance of logical information indicating that normal utilization of olive oil is effectively cardio defensive, just as assuming a job in diminishing the danger of significant maladies of the advanced world, for example, diabetes, certain tumors, and osteoporosis, and being related with expanded life span.

With regards to olive oil, the key is to purchase additional virgin so as to harvest full Sirtfood goodness. Virgin olive oil is acquired from the natural product exclusively by mechanical methods under conditions that don't prompt the crumbling of the oil, so you can be guaranteed of the quality and polyphenol content. "Additional virgin" alludes to the primary squeezing of the organic product ("virgin" is the subsequent squeezing); it has the best taste, quality, and Sirtfood certifications, and in this way is the one we emphatically suggest you use.

GARLIC

For a great many years garlic has been viewed as one of nature's miracle nourishments, with recuperating and reviving forces. Egyptians took care of garlic to pyramid teams to help their invulnerability and avoid different diseases, just as to improve their exhibition through its capacity to forestall weakness. Garlic is an amazing characteristic anti-toxin and antifungal regularly used to assist treat with tolerating ulcers. It can animate the lymphatic framework to "detox" by speeding up the expulsion of waste items from the body.

Furthermore, just as being examined for fat loss, it likewise sneaks up all of a sudden, bringing down cholesterol by around 10 percent and pulse by 5 to 7 percent, just as decreasing the tenacity of the blood and glucose levels.7 And on the off chance that you are stressed over that off-putting garlic scent, observe. At the point when ladies were solicited to evaluate a determination from men's stenches, those men who expended at least four cloves of garlic daily were decided to have a considerably more alluring and wonderful smell.8 Scientists trust it is on the grounds that it is seen as flagging better wellbeing. Furthermore, obviously, there are consistently mints for fresher breath! There is a stunt to getting greatest profit by eating garlic. The Sirtfood supplements in garlic are supplemented by another key supplement in it called allicin, which emits garlic's trademark fragrance. In any case, allicin just structures in garlic after physical "injury" to the bulb. What's more, its development is halted when presented to warm (cooking) or low pH (stomach corrosive). So while getting ready garlic, hack, mince, or pound, and afterward permit it to sit for around ten minutes to permit the allicin to shape before cooking or eating it.

GREEN TEA (PARTICULARLY MATCHA)

Green tea, the toast of the Orient, and always mainstream in the West, will be recognizable to many. As will the expanding consciousness of its medical advantages, connecting green tea utilization with less malignancy, coronary illness, diabetes, and osteoporosis. The explanation green tea is accepted to be so bravo is essentially because of its rich substance of a gathering of incredible plant mixes called catechins, the superstar being a specific sort of sirtuin-enacting catechin known as epigallocatechin gallate (EGCG).

Be that as it may, what's the entire whine about match? We like to consider match typical green tea on steroids. It is an exceptional powdered green tea that is set up by dissolving it straightforwardly in water, as opposed to regular green tea, which is set up as a mixture. The end result of devouring match is that it contains drastically more noteworthy degrees of the sirtuin-actuating compound

EGCG contrasted and different sorts of green tea. In case you're searching for additional support, Zen ministers depict match as "a definitive mental and clinical cure [which] can make one's life all the more full and complete."

KALE

We are pessimists on a fundamental level, so we are consistently wary of what's driving the most recent super food exposure fever. Is it science or is it personal stakes? Scarcely any nourishments have detonated on the wellbeing scene as of late as drastically as kale. Depicted as the "lean, green brassica sovereign" (alluding to its group of cruciferous vegetables), it has become the chic vegetable all wellbeing aficionados and foodies are gunning for.

There is even a National Kale Day every October. In any case, you don't need to hold up to that point to show your kale pride: there are Shirts as well, with in vogue mottos, for example, "Fueled by Kale" and "Roadway to Kale." For us, that is sufficient to set the alerts ringing.

Loaded up with doubts, we did the examination, and we need to concede that our decision is that kale does really merit its acclamations (in spite of the fact that we despite everything don't suggest the Shirts!). The explanation we are master kale is that it brags guard sums the sirtuin-actuating supplements quercetin and kaempferol, making it an absolute necessity remember for the Sirtfood Diet and the base of our Sirtfood green juice.

What's so invigorating about kale is that, dissimilar to the standard intriguing, hard to source, and excessively valued purported super nourishments; kale is accessible all over the place, privately developed, and truly reasonable.

MEDJOOL DATES

The incorporation of Medjool dates in a rundown of nourishments that invigorate weight loss and advances wellbeing may come as a shock—particularly when we reveal to you that Medjool dates contain a stunning 66 percent sugar. Sugar has no sirtuin-initiating properties at all; somewhat, it has settled connects to stoutness, coronary illness, and diabetes—a remarkable inverse of what we are hoping to accomplish. In any case, prepared and refined sugar is altogether different from sugar conveyed in a vehicle furnished essentially that is adjusted with sirtuin-initiating polyphenols: the Medjool date.

In complete complexity to typical sugar, Medjool dates, eaten with some restraint, really have no genuine recognizable glucose raising effects.9 actually; eating them is connected to having less diabetes and coronary illness. They have been a staple food around the globe for a considerable length of time, and lately there has been a blast of logical enthusiasm for dates, which sees them developing as a potential medication for various sicknesses.

Thus lays the uniqueness and intensity of the Sirtfood Diet: it invalidates the authoritative opinion and permits you to enjoy sweet things with some restraint without feeling regretful.

PARSLEY

Parsley is a culinary problem. It shows up so regularly in plans, yet so frequently it's the token green person. Best case scenario we serve a couple of twigs slashed up and hurled on a supper as an untimely idea, at the very least a lone branch only for ornamental purposes. In any case, it's regularly as yet mulling there on the plate long after we've completed the process of eating.

This culinary pigeonholing originates from its conventional use in old Rome as a trimming to eat after dinners to invigorate breathe, rather than being a piece of the feast itself. Furthermore, what a disgrace, since parsley is an incredible food pressing a lively and reviving taste that is loaded up with character

Taste aside, what makes parsley extremely uncommon is that it is a magnificent wellspring of the sirtuin-actuating supplement apigenin, a genuine aid given that it is once in a while found in critical amounts in different nourishments. Fascinatingly, apigenin ties to the benzodiazepine receptors in our cerebrums, helping us to unwind and supporting rest. Stack everything up, and it's time we acknowledged parsley not as universal food confetti however as a food in its own privilege so as to receive the great wellbeing rewards it can bring.

RED ENDIVE

To the extent vegetables go, endive is a moderately tenderfoot. Story has it that endive was found coincidentally by a Belgian rancher in 1830. The rancher put away chicory roots, and afterward utilized as a kind of espresso substitute, in his basement, just to disregard them. Upon his arrival he found that they had grown white leaves, which after tasting he saw as delicate, crunchy, and rather tasty.

Presently endive is developed everywhere throughout the world, including the US, and procures its Sirtfood identification on account of its great substance of the sirtuin activator lute Olin. What's more, notwithstanding the built up sirtuin-actuating benefits, lutein utilization has become a promising treatment approach for improving amiability in mentally unbalanced kids.

For those new to endive, it has a fresh surface and a sweet flavor joined by a mellow and wonderful sharpness. In case you're at any point adhered on the most proficient method to build endive in your diet, you can't lose by adding its leaves to a plate of mixed greens, where its welcome, tart flavor adds the ideal chomp to a fiery additional virgin olive oil–based dressing. Much the same as onion, red is ideal, however the yellow assortment can likewise be viewed as a Sirtfood. So while the red assortment can now and then be harder to find, you can have confidence that yellow is a totally appropriate other option.

RED ONIONS

Onions have been a dietary staple since the hour of our ancient ancestors, being probably the most punctual harvest to be developed, approximately 5,000 years back. With such a long history of utilization, and such powerful wellbeing giving properties, onions have been worshipped by numerous societies that have preceded us. The Egyptians held them specifically distinction as objects of love, in regards to their hover inside a-hover structure as emblematic of endless life. Furthermore, the Greeks accepted onions fortified competitors.

Prior to the Olympic Games, competitors would eat their way through huge measures of onions, in any event, drinking the juice! It's an extraordinary declaration to how significant antiquated dietary knowledge can be the point at which we consider that onions acquire their best twenty Sirtfood status since they are stuffed with the sirtuin-actuating compound quercetin—the extremely exacerbate that the universe of sports science has as of late started effectively looking into and promoting for improving games execution.

What's more, why red? Just on the grounds that they have the most noteworthy quercetin content, despite the fact that the standard yellow ones don't linger excessively far behind, and are a decent incorporation as well.

RED WINE

Any rundown of the best twenty Sirtfoods would not be finished without the consideration of red wine, the first Sirtfood. In the mid-1990s, the French Catch 22 stood out as truly newsworthy, with it being found that in spite of the French seeming to do everything incorrectly when it came to wellbeing (smoking, absence of activity, and utilization of rich food), they had lower passing rates from coronary illness than nations, for example, the US. Specialists proposed the explanation was the abundant measures of red wine expended. At that point in 1995, Danish specialists distributed work to demonstrate that low-to-direct red wine utilization decreased demise rates, while comparative liquor levels of brew had no impact and comparative liquor admissions of hard mixers expanded passing rates. In 2003, obviously, red wine's rich substance of a group of sirtuin-initiating supplements was revealed, and the rest, as is commonly said, became history.

Be that as it may, there's much more to red wine's noteworthy list of references. Red wine gives off an impression of being ready to avert the basic cold, with moderate wine consumers having a more prominent than 40 percent decrease in its incidence.12 Studies currently likewise show benefits for oral wellbeing and in counteraction of cavities.13 With moderate utilization additionally appeared to build social holding and out-of-the-case thinking, that after-work drink among associates to examine work ventures seems to have an establishing in solid science.

Obviously, balance is critical. Just limited quantities are required for advantage, and abundance liquor rapidly fixes the great. The sweet spot has all the earmarks of being staying inside US rules of up to one 5-ounce drink every day for ladies and up to two 5-ounce drinks every day for men. To guarantee greatest sirtuin initiating value for your money, wines from the New York district (particularly pinot noir, cabernet sauvignon, and merlot) have the most noteworthy polyphenol substance of the most broadly accessible wines.

SOY

Soy items have a long history as a vital piece of the diet of numerous Asia Pacific nations, for example, China, Japan, and the Koreas. Analysts initially got went on to soy after the perception that high soy–devouring nations had uniquely lower paces of specific malignant growths, particularly of the bosom and prostate. This is believed to be because of an uncommon gathering of polyphenols contained inside soybeans known as is avones, which can well change how estrogens work in the body, and incorporate the sirtuin-activators daidzein and formononetin. Utilization of soy items has likewise been connected to a decrease in the frequency or seriousness of an assortment of conditions, for example, cardiovascular illness, menopausal manifestations, and bone loss.

Exceptionally handled, supplement stripped types of soybean are currently an omnipresent fixing added to many prepared food items. The advantages are just harvested through regular soy items, for example, tofu, an incredible vegetarian protein source, or in a matured structure, for example, tempeh, natto, or our top pick, miso, a customary Japanese glue aged with a normally happening parasite that outcomes in an extraordinary umami flavor.

STRAWBERRIES

Natural product has been progressively attacked as of late, getting negative criticism in the developing intensity against sugar. Luckily for berry sweethearts, such an insulted notoriety couldn't be all the more badly merited. While all berries are nutritional powerhouses, strawberries win their best twenty Sirtfood status because of their plenitude of the sirtuin activator setin. Furthermore, concentrates currently embrace eating strawberries consistently to advance healthy maturing, fighting off Alzheimer's, malignant growth, diabetes, coronary illness, and osteoporosis. Concerning their sugar content, it's low, a unimportant teaspoon of sugar per 31/2 ounces.

Intriguingly, just as being characteristically low in sugar those, strawberries effect sly affect improving how the body handles starches. What specialists have found is that adding strawberries to starches has the impact of diminishing insulin request, basically transforming the food into a supported vitality releaser. What's more, new research is presently proposing that eating strawberries has comparative impacts to sedate treatment in diabetes treatment. The extraordinary seventeenth-century doctor William Head servant wrote in commendation of the strawberry: "Without a doubt God could have improved a berry, yet surely God never did." We can just concur.

TURMERIC

Turmeric, a cousin of ginger, is the tenderfoot in food patterns, with Google naming it the "breakout star" element of 2015. In spite of the fact that here in the West we are just going to it now, it has been acknowledged in Asia for a large number of years for both culinary and clinical reasons

 Fantastically, India creates almost the whole world's flexibly of turmeric, devouring 80 percent of it itself. Alongside the advantages of the "brilliant zest" we saw on pages 60–61, turmeric is utilized in Asia to treat skin conditions, for example, skin inflammation, psoriasis, dermatitis, and rash. Prior to Indian weddings, a service happens where turmeric glue is applied to lady of the hour and husband to be as a skin marvel routine yet in addition to represent averting detestable.

Something that limits the adequacy of turmeric is that its key sirtuin-enacting supplement, curcumin, is ineffectively consumed by the body when we eat it. Notwithstanding, look into shows that we can beat this by cooking it in fluid, including fat, and including dark pepper, all of which drastically increment its assimilation. This fits impeccably with conventional Indian cooking, where it is normally joined with ghee and dark pepper in curries and other hot dishes, and confirmation again that science is just barely finding the well-established shrewdness of customary methods of eating.

PECANS

Dating right back to 7000 BCE, pecans are the most seasoned tree food known to man, beginning in old Persia, where they were the save of sovereignty. Quick forward to today and pecans are a US example of overcoming adversity. California drives the way, with the Focal Valley of California prestigious for being the prime pecan developing district. California pecans give 99 percent of the business gracefully to the US and a stunning three-quarter of pecan exchange around the world.

As per the Maritime framework, which positions nourishments as indicated by how healthy they are and has been supported by the American School of Preventive Medication; pecans lead the path as the main nut for wellbeing. However, what truly makes pecans stand apart for us is the manner by which they y despite regular reasoning: they are high in fat and calories, yet entrenched for decreasing weight and slicing the danger of metabolic maladies, for example, cardiovascular infection and diabetes. That is the intensity of sirtuin enactment.

Less notable, however similarly charming, is the developing exploration demonstrating pecans to be a ground-breaking hostile to maturing food. Just as forestalling the decrease in physical capacity with age, inquire about additionally focuses to their advantages as a cerebrum food with the possibility to hinder mind maturing and lessen the danger of degenerative mind issue.

CHAPTER NINE: PHASE 1: 7 POUNDS IN SEVEN DAYS

Welcome to Stage 1 of the Sirtfood Diet. This is the hyper-achievement stage, where you will step toward accomplishing a slimmer and more slender body. Follow our basic bit by bit directions and utilize the flavorful plans accommodated you. Notwithstanding our standard seven-day plan, we additionally have a without meat variant, which is reasonable for the two veggie lovers and vegetarians. Don't hesitate to go with whichever one you like.

WHAT'S IN STORE

During Stage 1, you will receive the full rewards of our clinically demonstrated strategy for shedding 7 pounds in seven days. Be that as it may, recollect this incorporates muscle gain, so don't get hung up absolutely with the numbers on the scales (see pages 35–36). Nor should you start gauging yourself day by day. Truth is told, we regularly observe the scales sneaking up over the most recent couple of long stretches of Stage 1 because of muscle gain, while waistlines keep on contracting.

That is the reason we need you to take a gander at the scales, yet not be administered by them. Look at what you look like in the mirror, how your garments are fitting, or whether you have to move a score on your belt. These are for the most part incredible markers of the more pound changes in your body organization.

Know about different changes as well, for example, in your feeling of prosperity, your vitality levels, and how clear your skin looks. You can even get estimations of your general cardiovascular and metabolic wellbeing performed at your nearby drug store to see changes in things like your pulse, glucose levels, and blood fats, for example, cholesterol and triglycerides. Keep in mind, weight loss aside, the presentation of Sirtfoods into your diet is a gigantic advance in making your cells fitter and progressively impervious to ailment, setting you up for a lifetime of excellent wellbeing.

STEP BY STEP INSTRUCTIONS TO FOLLOW STAGE 1

To make Stage 1 as plain cruising as could reasonably be expected, we'll direct you through the total seven-day plan each day in turn, including the lowdown on the Sirtfood green juice and simple to- follow, delightful plans at all times.

Stage 1 of the Sirtfood Diet depends on two particular stages:

Days 1 to 3 are the most serious, and during this period you can eat up to a furthest reaches of 1,000 calories every day, comprising of:-

- 3 x Sirtfood green juice

- 1 x primary feast

Days 4 to 7 will see your food consumption increment to a furthest reaches of 1,500 calories every day, comprising of:

- 2 x Sirtfood green juices

- 2 x fundamental dinners

There are not many standards for following the diet. At last it's tied in with fitting it into your lifestyle and around everyday living for delayed achievement. Be that as it may, here are a couple of basic yet huge effect tips for accomplishing the best result:

1. Get a Decent Juicer: Squeezing is a vital piece of the Sirtfood Diet, and a juicer is probably the best venture you will make for your wellbeing. While financial plan ought to be the deciding component, a few juicers are progressively viable at separating the juice from green verdant vegetables and herbs, with the

Beeville brand being among the best of the normally accessible juicers we have attempted.

2. Preparation Is Vital: From the abundance of criticism we have made them thing, is clear: the individuals who arranged ahead of time were the best. Get acquainted with the fixings and plans and stock up on what you need. With everything composed and prepared, you'll be astounded at how simple the entire procedure is.

3. Save Time: On the off chance that you are tight for time, get ready keenly. Dinners can be made the prior night. Juices can be made in mass, and kept in the ice chest for as long as three days (or longer in the cooler) before their degrees of sirtuin actuating supplements begin to drop. Simply shield it from light, and possibly include the match when you are prepared to expend it.

4. Eat Early: It is smarter to eat prior in the day, and suppers and juices ought to in a perfect world not be devoured later than 7 p.m.; in any case the diet is intended to t with your lifestyle, and late eaters despite everything receive incredible reward.

5. Space out the Juices: To upgrade assimilation of the green juices, they ought to be expended at any rate an hour prior or two hours after a supper and spread out for the duration of the day, instead of having them excessively near one another.

6. Eat until Fulfilled: Sirtfoods can effect sly affect craving and a few people will be full before completing their dinners. Tune in to your body and eat until you are fulfilled as opposed to compelling all the food down.

7. Enjoy the Excursion: Don't get up to speed with the ultimate objective; rather remain aware of the excursion. This diet is tied in with commending food

in the entirety of its miracle, for its medical advantages yet similarly for the delight and happiness it brings. Research shows that when we keep our brains concentrated on the way rather than the goal, we are significantly more liable to succeed.

WHAT TO DRINK

Just as the suggested day by day servings of green juices, you can expend different liquids openly all through Stage 1. These ought to be no caloric beverages, ideally plain water, dark espresso, and green tea. On the off chance that your typical preference is for dark or home grown teas, don't hesitate to incorporate these too.

Soda pops and organic product juices are abandoned. Rather, on the off chance that you need to jazz things up, have a go at adding some cut strawberries to at present or shining water to make your own Sirtfood implanted wellbeing drink. Save it in the cooler for two or three hours and you'll have a wonderfully reviving option in contrast to soda pops and squeezes?

One thing to know about is that we don't prescribe unexpected enormous changes to your ordinary espresso utilization. Caffeine withdrawal manifestations can cause you to feel lousy for several days; similarly, enormous increments can be disagreeable for those especially delicate with the impacts of caffeine. We likewise suggest that espresso be smashed dark, without including milk, since certain analysts have discovered that the option of milk can decrease the retention of the useful sirtuin-initiating nutrients.[1] The equivalent has been found for green tea,[2] however including some lemon squeeze really expands the ingestion of its sirtuin-enacting supplements.

Do recollect this is the hyper-achievement stage, and keeping in mind that you ought to be support by the way that it is for multi week just, you do should be more trained. During the current week we incorporate liquor, as red wine, yet just as a cooking fixing.

THE SIRTFOOD GREEN JUICE

The green juice is a fundamental piece of Stage 1 of the Sirtfood Diet. All the fixings are amazing Sirtfoods, and in every juice you get a strong mixed drink of normal mixes, for example, apigenin, kaempferol, lutein, quercetin, and EGCG that cooperate to turn on your sirtuin qualities and advance fat loss. To that we've included lemon, as its regular sharpness has been appeared to ensure, balance out, and increment the retention of the beverage's sirtuin-actuating supplements. We've likewise included a dash of apple and ginger for taste. Both of these are in this manner discretionary. To be sure, numerous individuals find that once they are acquainted with the flavor of the juice, they forget about the apple inside and out.

SIRTFOOD GREEN JUICE (SERVES 1)

2 huge bunches (around 21/2 ounces or 75g) kale a huge bunch (1 ounce or 30g) arugula a little bunch (around 1/4 ounce or 5g) at-leaf parsley 2 to 3 enormous celery stems (51/2 ounces or 150g), including leaves

1/2 medium green apple

1/2-to 1-inch (1 to 2.5 cm) bit of new ginger juice of 1/2 lemon

1/2 level teaspoon match powder

Days 1 to 3 of Stage 1: added distinctly to the initial two juices of the day; Days 4 to 7 of Stage 1: added to the two juices

Note that while in our pilot preliminary all amounts were weighed out precisely as recorded, our experience is that bunch estimates work very well. Truth be told, they better tailor the supplement amount to a person's body size. Bigger people will in general have bigger hands and subsequently get a relatively higher measure of Sirtfood supplements to coordinate their body size, and the other way around for littler individuals.

Mix the greens (kale, arugula, and parsley) together, and

afterward squeeze them. We find that juicers can truly vary in their effectiveness at squeezing verdant vegetables, and you may need to rejuice the leftovers before proceeding onward to different fixings. The objective is to wind up with around 2 liquid ounces or near 1/4 cup (50ml) of juice from the greens.

☐ Now juice the celery, apple, and ginger.

☐ You can strip the lemon and put it through the juicer also, however we find it a lot simpler to just press the lemon by hand into the juice. By this stage, you ought to have around 1 cup (250ml) of juice altogether, maybe marginally more.

☐ It is just when the juice is made and prepared to serve that you include the match. Pour a limited quantity of the juice into a glass, at that point include the match and mix energetically with a fork or teaspoon. We just use match in the initial two beverages of the day since it contains moderate measures of caffeine (a similar substance as an ordinary cup of tea). For individuals not accustomed to it, it might keep them alert whenever alcoholic late.

Once the match is broken up, include the rest of the juice. Give it a mix, at that point your juice is prepared to drink. Don't hesitate to top up with plain water, as indicated by taste.

STAGE 1: YOUR SEVEN-DAY GUIDE

If it's not too much troubles note that you have to peruse the formula notes on before starting to cook.

For quite a long time 1 to 3, take the juices at independent times (e.g., before anything else, midmorning, and midafternoon), and select one of the norm or veggie lover feast alternatives and eat it during a period that suits you (as a rule had for lunch or supper).

DAY 1

On Day 1, you will expend:

- [ ] 3 x Sirtfood green juices

- [ ] 1 x fundamental feast (standard or vegetarian choice), either:

Asian shrimp pan sear with buckwheat noodles + 1/2 to 3/4 ounce (15 to 20g) dull chocolate (85 percent cocoa solids) or Miso and sesame coated tofu with ginger and bean stew pan-seared greens (veggie lover) + 1/2 to 3/4 ounce (15 to 20g) dim chocolate (85 percent cocoa solids)

DAY 2

On Day 2, you will devour:

- [ ] 3 x Sirtfood green juices

- [ ] 1 x principle feast (standard or veggie lover alternative), either:

Turkey escalope with sage, tricks, and parsley and spiced caulis blossom "couscous" + 1/2 to 3/4 ounce (15 to 20g) dull chocolate (85 percent cocoa solids) or Kale and red onion dal with buckwheat (veggie lover) + 1/2 to 3/4 ounce (15 to 20g) dim chocolate (85 percent cocoa solids)

DAY 3

On Day 3, you will devour:

- [ ] 3 x Sirtfood green juice
- [ ] 1 x principle dinner (standard or veggie lover choice), either:

Sweet-smelling chicken bosom with kale and red onions and a tomato and bean stew salsa + 1/2 to 3/4 ounce (15 to 20g) dim chocolate (85 percent cocoa solids) or Harissa prepared tofu with caulis bloom "couscous" (vegetarian) + 1/2 to 3/4 ounce (15 to 20g) dull chocolate (85 percent cocoa solids)

For a considerable length of time 4 to 7, take the juices at discrete times (e.g., the primary squeeze either before anything else or midmorning, the second squeeze midafternoon); select your suppers from either the norm or veggie lover alternatives, and eat them during a period that suits you (as a rule had for breakfast/lunch and supper). Additionally, as per your hunger, you may keep on including 1/2 to 3/4 ounce (15 to 20g) dim chocolate (85 percent cocoa solids) every day, at your attentiveness.

DAY 4

On Day 4, you will devour:

- 2 x Sirtfood green juices

- 2 x principle dinners (standard or vegetarian choice), either:

Supper 1: Sirt muesli

Supper 2: Seared salmon filet with caramelized endive, arugula, and celery leaf plate of mixed greens or
Supper 1: Sirt muesli (vegetarian) Supper 2: Tuscan bean stew (vegetarian) **DAY 5**
On Day 5, you will devour:

- 2 x Sirtfood green juices

- 2 x primary dinners (standard or vegetarian choice), either: Supper 1: Strawberry buckwheat Supper 2: Miso-marinated heated cod with sautéed greens and sesame or Supper 1: Strawberry buckwheat (vegetarian)
Supper 2: Soba (buckwheat noodles) in a miso stock with tofu, celery, and kale (vegetarian)

DAY 6

On Day 6, you will expend:

☐ 2 x Sirtfood green juices

☐ 2 x principle dinners (standard or vegetarian alternative), either: Supper 1: Sirt super serving of mixed greens
Supper 2: Burn barbecued hamburger with a red wine jus, onion rings, garlic kale, and herb-broiled potatoes
Or on the other hand Feast 1: Lentil Sirt super serving of mixed greens (veggie lover) Feast 2: Kidney bean mole with prepared potato (veggie lover)

DAY 7

On Day 7, you will expend:

☐ 2 x Sirtfood green juices

☐ 2 x principle suppers (standard or veggie lover choice), either: Supper 1: Sirtfood omelet
Supper 2: Prepared chicken bosom with pecan and parsley pesto and red onion plate of mixed greens or
Supper 1: Potato plate of mixed greens (vegan)

Supper 2: Broiled eggplant wedges with pecan and parsley pesto and tomato plate of mixed greens (veggie lover)

CHAPTER TEN: PHASE 2: MAINTENANCE

Congrats on finishing Stage 1 of the Sirtfood Diet! As of now you ought to be seeing extraordinary outcomes with fat loss and are looking slimmer and increasingly conditioned, however feeling revived and reenergized. Things being what they are, what now?

Having seen these regularly astounding changes ourselves firsthand, we realize the amount you'll need to save every one of those advantages, however observe stunningly better outcomes. All things considered, Sirtfoods are intended to be eaten forever. The inquiry is the way you adjust what you have been doing in Stage 1 into your standard dietary everyday practice.

That is actually what incited us to make a subsequent fourteen-day support plan intended to assist you with making the change from Stage 1 to your progressively ordinary dietary daily practice and in this way help continue and further broaden the advantages of the Sirtfood Diet.

WHAT'S IN STORE

During Stage 2, you will solidify your weight-loss results and keep on consistently get more fit. Recollect that the one striking thing we have found with the Sirtfood Diet is that most or the entirety of the weight that individuals lose is from fat, and that numerous really put on some muscle. So we need to remind you again not to pass judgment on your advancement simply by the numbers on the scale. Glance in the mirror to check whether you are looking more slender and progressively conditioned, perceive how your garments are fitting, and drink up the commendations that you will get from others.

Recollect excessively that similarly as the weight loss will proceed, the medical advantages will develop. By following the fourteen-day support plan, you're truly beginning to set out the establishments for a fate of lifelong wellbeing.

THE MOST EFFECTIVE METHOD TO FOLLOW STAGE 2

The way to accomplishment in this stage is to continue pressing your diet loaded with Sirtfoods. To make it as simple as could be expected under the circumstances, we've assembled a seven-day menu plan for you to follow, including scrumptious family-accommodating plans, with every day pressed to the rafters with Sirtfoods for guidance in regards to youngsters). You should simply rehash the seven-day plan twice to finish the fourteen days of Stage 2.

On every one of the fourteen days your diet will comprise of:

- 3 x adjusted Sirtfood-rich dinners

- 1 x Sirtfood green juice

- 1 to 2 x discretionary Sirtfood nibble snacks

Indeed, there are no unbending guidelines for when you need to devour these. Be adaptable and t them around your day. Two straightforward dependable guidelines are:

- Have your green squeeze either before anything else, at any rate thirty minutes before breakfast or midmorning.
- Try your best to eat your night dinner by 7 p.m.

PART SIZES

Our concentration during Stage 2 isn't on checking calories. Over the drawn out this is definitely not a commonsense or even fruitful methodology for the normal individual. Rather we're concentrating on reasonable segments, truly even dinners, and generally significant, topping off on Sirtfoods so you can keep on profiting by their fat consuming and wellbeing advancing impacts.

We have likewise developed the suppers in the arrangement to make them satisfying, which will assist you with feeling full for more. That, joined with the normal hunger directing impacts of Sirtfoods, implies that you won't go through the following fourteen days feeling hungry, yet rather agreeably fulfilled, very much took care of, and amazingly all around supported.

Similarly as in Stage 1, make sure to tune in to your body and be guided by your hunger. On the off chance that you get ready suppers as indicated by our directions and discover you are easily full before you've completed a feast, at that point it's consummately ne to quit eating!

WHAT TO DRINK

You will keep on including one green squeeze day by day all through Stage 2. This is to keep you beat up with elevated levels of Sirtfoods.

Similarly as in Stage 1, you can devour different liquids unreservedly all through Stage 2. Our favored beverages for you to incorporate stay plain water, custom made enhanced water, espresso, and green tea. On the off chance that your inclination is for dark or white tea, don't hesitate to appreciate. The equivalent applies to home grown teas. The best news is that you can appreciate the incidental glass of red wine during Stage 2. Red wine is a Sirtfood because of its substance of sirtuin- enacting polyphenols, particularly resveratrol and piceatannol, settling on it by a long shot the best decision of mixed refreshment. Be that as it may, with liquor itself effect sly affecting our fat cells, balance is still best, and all through Stage 2 we prescribe constraining your admission to one glass of red wine with a feast, on a few days out of each week.

COMING BACK TO THREE SUPPERS

During Stage 1 you expended only a couple of suppers daily, which gave you heaps of edibility over when you ate your dinners. As we currently come back to an increasingly typical daily practice and the time-demonstrated example of three suppers per day, it's a decent time to discuss breakfast. Having a decent breakfast sets us up for the afternoon, expanding our vitality and focus levels. As far as our digestion, eating prior keeps our glucose and fat levels in line. That morning meal is something to be thankful for is borne out by various examinations that ordinarily show that individuals who consistently have breakfast are less inclined to be overweight.

The explanation behind this is because of our inward body timekeepers. Our bodies anticipate that us should eat from the get-go fully expecting when we will be generally dynamic and requiring fuel. However on some random day, upwards of 33% of us will skip breakfast. It's an exemplary manifestation of our bustling present day lives, and the recognition is that there basically isn't sufficient opportunity to eat well. Be that as it may, as you will see, with the clever morning meals we have spread out for you here, nothing could be further from reality.

Regardless of whether it's the Sirtfood smoothie that can be flushed in a hurry, the premade Sirt muesli, or the brisk and simple Sirtfood fried eggs/tofu, finding those additional couple of moments in the first part of the day will procure profits for your day as well as for your more extended term weight and wellbeing.

With Sirtfoods attempting to supercharge our vitality levels, there is much more to be picked up from getting an early morning hit of them to begin your day. This is accomplished through having a Sirtfood-rich breakfast, yet particularly through the consideration of the green juice, which we suggest you have either before anything else—in any event thirty minutes before breakfast — or midmorning. From our own clinical experience, we do get numerous reports of individuals who drink their green squeeze first thing and don't feel hungry for a few hours thereafter.

In the event that this is the impact it has on you, it is impeccably ne to hold up two or three hours before eating. Simply don't skip it. On the other hand, you can commence your day with a decent breakfast, and afterward hold up a few hours before having the green juice. Be adaptable and simply go with whatever works for you.

SIRTFOOD NIBBLES

With regards to eating, you can accept the only choice available. There has been such a great amount of discussion about in the case of eating continuous, littler suppers is best for weight loss, or whether you should simply adhere to three adjusted dinners daily. In all actuality, it doesn't generally make a difference.

The manner in which we have built the upkeep menu for you guarantees you will eat three even Sirtfood-rich suppers every day, and you may discover you truly needn't bother with a tidbit. In any case, maybe you've been occupied in the of face, working out, or running around with the children, and need something to hold you over to the following supper. Furthermore, if that "small something" is going to give you a whammy of Sirtfood supplements and taste heavenly, at that point it's glad days. This is the reason we made our "Sirtfood chomps." These shrewd little bites are a really faultless treat made completely from Sirtfoods: dates, pecans, cocoa, additional virgin olive oil, and turmeric. For the days you need them, we suggest eating one, or a limit of two, every day. **"SIRTIFYING" YOUR DINNERS**

We've seen that the main economical diets are ones of consideration, not rejection. Be that as it may, genuine progress goes past this—the diet must be perfect with advanced living. Regardless of whether it is the comfort to satisfy the needs of our furious lives or fitting in with our job as the bon vivant at evening gatherings, the manner in which we eat ought to be without bother. You ought to have the option to make the most of your smooth figure and brilliant sparkle, rather than stressing over silly food requests and limitations.

What's so phenomenal about Sirtfoods is that they are extremely available, recognizable, and simple to remember for your diet. Here, as you overcome any barrier between Stage 1 and routine eating, you will fabricate establishments for another, improved method of lifelong eating.

The key guideline is the thing that we call "Sirtifying" your dinners. This is the place we take natural dishes, including numerous exemplary top picks, and with some sharp trades and basic Sirtfood considerations we keep all the incredible taste however include a ton more goodness. All through Stage 2 you will see exactly how effectively this is accomplished.

Models incorporate our delectable Sirtfood smoothie for the ideal in a hurry breakfast in a period starved world and the basic change from wheat to buckwheat for adding additional taste and zoom to the much-cherished solace food that is pasta. Then notorious, dearest dishes, for example, stew con carne and curry don't require a lot of progress, with the customary plans offering Sirtfood bonanzas. Furthermore, who said inexpensive food implied terrible food? We consolidate the credible energetic kinds of a pizza and expel the blame when you make it yourself.

There's no compelling reason to express goodbye to extravagance either, as demonstrated by our flapjacks covered with berries and dull chocolate sauce. It's not even sweet, its morning meal, and it's incredible for you. Straightforward changes: you keep on eating the nourishments you love while driving a healthy weight and prosperity. What's more, that is the dietary unrest that is Sirtfoods.

COOKING FOR ADDITIONAL

To grasp this, we are presently entering a "Sirtfoods for all" stage, where plans start to take into account a larger number of mouths than one. Regardless of whether it is for family or companions, the new supper plans just as the Sirtfood-pressed soup we present in this stage are planned considering cooking for four. Also, for those as yet cooking for a couple of, why not exploit preparing cluster suppers for freezing to have dinners prepared for one week from now?

FOURTEEN-DAY DINNER PLAN

Notwithstanding our standard arrangement, we additionally have a sans meat form, which is appropriate for the two veggie lovers and vegetarians. Don't hesitate to go with whichever one you like, or even blend and match. Every day you will devour:

☐ 1 x Sirtfood green juice

☐ 3 x principle dinners (standard or vegetarian choices, see next page)

☐ 1 to 2 x discretionary Sirtfood chomps

Devour the juice either before anything else, at any rate thirty minutes before breakfast, or midmorning.

CHAPTER ELEVEN: SIRTFOODS FOR LIFE

Congrats, you've presently completed the two periods of the Sirtfood Diet! Allows simply check out what you've accomplished. You've finished the hyper-achievement stage, encountering in the district of 7 pounds of weight loss, which likely incorporates some alluring muscle gain.

You've merged that weight loss and further improved your body creation all through the fourteen- day upkeep stage.

Generally significant, you've denoted the start of your very own wellbeing upheaval. You have stood firm against the tide of sick wellbeing that so frequently strikes as we get more established. Expanded vitality, essentialness, and prosperity are simply the future you have picked.

At this point you will be acquainted with the best twenty Sirtfoods and have increased a valuation for exactly how incredible they are. Not just that, you will likewise have gotten very proficient at incorporating and getting a charge out of them in your diet. It is basic that these nourishments stay a conspicuous component in your everyday eating schedule, for the proceeded with weight loss and prosperity they bring. Yet at the same time, they are just twenty nourishments and, all things too much of the same thing will drive a person crazy. So what next?

In this part we give you the outline for lifelong wellbeing. It's tied in with getting your body in ideal offset with a diet that is reasonable and manageable for all, and gives all the wellbeing improving supplements we need. It's tied in with proceeding to receive the weight-loss benefits of the Sirtfood Diet utilizing the absolute best nourishments that nature brings to the table.

PAST THE MAIN TWENTY SIRTFOODS

We've seen why Sirtfoods are so useful: certain plants have refined pressure reaction frameworks that produce exacerbates that initiate sirtuins—a similar fat-consuming and life span framework in the body that is enacted by fasting and exercise. The more noteworthy the measure of these aggravates that plants delivers in light of pressure, the more noteworthy the advantage we get from eating them. Our rundown of the best twenty Sirtfoods is comprised of the nourishments that truly stand apart by uprightness of being particularly pressed brimming with these mixes, and in this manner the nourishments that have the most excellent capacity to affect body arrangement and prosperity. However the sirtuin-enacting impact of nourishments isn't a win big or bust guideline. There are numerous different plants out there that produce moderate degrees of sirtuin-actuating supplements, and we urge you to truly extend the assortment and decent variety of your diet by eating these generously as well. The Sirtfood Diet is about consideration and the more prominent the assortment of nourishments with sirtuin actuating properties that can be fused into the diet, the better. Particularly if that implies including much a greater amount of your preferred nourishments to maximize the joy and satisfaction you can harvest from your dinners.

How about we utilize the relationship of activity. The best twenty Sirtfoods are the (substantially more pleasurable) likeness working it out in the rec center, with Stage 1 being the "training camp." conversely, eating those different nourishments with progressively moderate degrees of sirtuin- initiating supplements resembles receiving the benefits of going out for a decent walk. Contrast that with the ordinary diet with sustenance esteem proportional to lying on the lounge chair sitting in front of the television throughout the day. Without a doubt, working it out in the exercise center is acceptable, however you'll before long get tired of that if that is everything you do. That walk ought to be supported as well, particularly in the event that it implies you are not deciding to lie on the lounge chair.

For instance, we remembered strawberries for our main twenty

Sirtfoods on the grounds that they are the most outstanding wellspring of the sirtuin activator setin. However on the off chance that we look all the more extensively at berries as a nutritional category, we find that they have benefits for metabolic wellbeing just as advancing healthy maturing. Auditing their nutritional synthesis, we locate that different berries, for example, blackberries, dark currants, blueberries, and raspberries likewise have eminent degrees of sirtuin enacting supplements.

The equivalent applies to nuts. Notwithstanding their calorie content, so valuable are nuts that they really advance weight loss and help move creeps from the midsection. This is notwithstanding cutting the danger of incessant infection. While pecans are our hero nut, sirtuin-actuating supplements are likewise found in chestnuts, walnuts, pistachios, and even peanuts.

At that point we change our consideration regarding grains. There has been a developing abhorrence for grains as of late in certain quarters. However examines interface entire grain utilization to decrease inflammation, diabetes, coronary illness, and malignancy. While they don't match the Sirtfood certifications of the pseudo-grain buckwheat, we do see the nearness of noteworthy sirtuin-initiating supplements in other entire grains. What's more, obviously, when entire grains are prepared into refined "white" forms, their sirtuin-initiating supplement content is demolished. These refined adaptations are a remarkable poisonous bundle, and are involved in a plenty of cutting edge wellbeing pains. We're not saying that you can never eat them, but instead that you will be vastly improved off staying with the entire grain form at whatever point you can. For the individuals who need to remain sans gluten, quinoa is a decent Sirtfood alternative. What's more, for an incredible entire grain Sirtfood nibble cherished by all, look no farther than popcorn. Indeed, even notorious "super nourishments" get in on the demonstration with any semblance of goji berries and chia seeds having Sirtfood properties. This is most likely the accidental explanation behind their watched medical advantages. While it implies they are in reality bravo to eat, we additionally know there are less expensive, increasingly open, and better choices out there, so don't feel constrained to get on board with that specific fleeting trend. We see this equivalent example across numerous nutritional categories.

Obviously, these are typically the nourishments that science has set up are beneficial for us and that we ought to eat a greater amount of. Underneath we have recorded an extra forty nourishments that we have found likewise have Sirtfood properties. To keep up and proceed with your weight loss and prosperity, we effectively urge you to incorporate these nourishments as you truly grow the collection of your diet.

VEGETABLES

- Artichokes
- Asparagus

- Bok

- Broccoli

- Green beans

- Shallots

- Watercress

- White onions

- Yellow endive

ORGANIC PRODUCTS

- Apples

- Blackberries

- Black currants

- Black plums

- Cranberries

- Goji berries

- Kumquats

- Raspberries

- Red grapes

NUTS AND SEEDS

- Chestnuts

- Chia seeds

- Peanuts

- Pecan nuts

- Pistachio nuts

- Sun bloom seeds

GRAINS AND PSEUDO-GRAINS

- Popcorn

- ☐ Quinoa

- ☐ Whole-wheat our

BEANS

- ☐ Fava beans

- ☐ White beans (e.g., cannellini or naval force)

HERBS AND FLAVORS

- ☐ Chives

- ☐ Cinnamon

- ☐ Dill (new and dried)

- ☐ Dried oregano

- ☐ Dried sage

- ☐ Ginger

- ☐ Peppermint (new and dried)

- ☐ Thyme (new and dried)

REFRESHMENTS

- ☐ Black tea

- ☐ White tea

PROTEIN

A high-protein diet is one of the most advanced diets of ongoing years. The utilization of higher measures of protein when dieting has been found to advance satiety, look after digestion, and decrease loss of bulk. In any case, it's when Sirtfoods are joined with protein that things get taken to an unheard of level. As you may review, protein is a fundamental incorporation in a Sirtfood-based diet to receive greatest rewards. Protein is comprised of amino acids, and it is a particular amino corrosive, leucine, that intensely supplements the activities of Sirtfoods, improving their belongings. It does this basically by changing our phone condition so that the sirtuin-actuating supplements from our diet work substantially more viably. This implies we get the best result from a Sirtfood-rich feast that is joined with leucine-rich protein. The best dietary wellsprings of leucine incorporate red meat, poultry, fish, fish, eggs, and dairy.

CREATURE BASED PROTEIN

As of late creature items have been ensnared as a contributing reason for some Western maladies, particularly malignant growth. On the off chance that that genuinely is the situation, eating them with Sirtfoods probably won't appear to be such a splendid thought. So as to let that go, here's our lowdown.

One of the huge worries about dairy is that it's a straightforward food as well as an exceptionally advanced flagging framework for initiating fast body growth in posterity. While this has an esteemed reason in early life, in grown-up life it may not be so fitting. Industrious and hyper initiation of the key growth signal that dairy triggers in the body (called mTOR) is currently connected with maturing and the improvement old enough related issue, for example, heftiness, type 2 diabetes, malignancy, and neurodegenerative diseases.1 In spite of the fact that the complexities of this flagging framework are a generally new region of research so still especially an obscure and hypothetical hazard, this loans approval to why individuals would avoid dairy items. Be that as it may, there is one thing research focuses to: in the event that we add Sirtfoods to a diet containing dairy, they repress the improper impacts of mTOR on our cells, cancelling this hazard, making Sirtfoods an absolute necessity incorporate with a dairy-based diet.

In general, surveys of the connection among dairy and malignant growth are blended. At the point when we stack up all the examination, with regards to a Sirtfood-rich diet, moderate dairy utilization is impeccably ne and can offer numerous important supplements to supplement Sirtfoods.

Just as being a significant protein source, dairy is a magnificent wellspring of nutrients and minerals, for example, iodine, calcium, and phosphorus. Our proposal for grown-ups is to devour up to three servings of dairy (yet close to around 1 quart [1 liter] of milk, or proportional) a day.

While proof involving them in bosom and prostate malignant growth is entirely slight on the ground, there is real worry that red and prepared meat utilization assumes a job in inside cancer. Handled meat, for example, ham, wieners, and pepperoni. While there is no compelling reason to strike it off the menu totally, it ought to be remembered for simply modest quantities as opposed to being a staple.

The uplifting news about red meat is that exploration shows that cooking it with Sirtfoods revokes its malignant growth hazard, regardless of whether it be making a marinade with herbs, flavors, and additional virgin olive oil; cooking your problem with onions; or basically including a pleasant cup of green tea to the feast or enjoying after-supper dull chocolate. These all sneak up suddenly that really assists with killing red meat's unsafe impacts. While we are in support of having your steak and eating it, don't go over the edge. Red meat admission is best kept beneath around 1 pound (500g) every week (cooked weight), which is generally what might be compared to 1.5 pounds (700 to 750g) crude.

Poultry is an astounding wellspring of protein, alongside nutrients and minerals, for example, B nutrients, potassium, and phosphorus. Our suggestion for grown-ups is to eat it unreservedly. Red meat is additionally a fantastic wellspring of protein, alongside nutrients and minerals, for example, iron, zinc, and nutrient B. Our proposal for grown-ups is to eat up to a limit of three servings every week.

The connection between egg utilization and disease hazard has not been concentrated as completely as meat and dairy items have, yet in such manner there appears to be little purpose behind concern. Rather, what eggs have been embroiled in causing is coronary illness. This is on the grounds that they are a significant wellspring of dietary cholesterol. Along these lines we are advised to constrain egg utilization.

Curiously, different nations, including Nepal, Thailand, and South Africa, suggest devouring eggs as regularly as consistently for their nutritional advantages. So who is correct? The proof is persuading in agreeing with the last mentioned. Every day egg utilization isn't connected to any expanded danger of coronary illness or stroke. While explicit hereditary conditions may require decreased dietary cholesterol consumption, for everyone this limitation isn't important.

Just as being a significant protein source, eggs are a superb wellspring of fundamental supplements, for example, B nutrients, nutrient an, and carotenoids. Our suggestion for grown-ups is to eat as wanted as a feature of a decent diet.

THE INTENSITY OF THREE

The second significant supplement bunch that effectively supplements Sirtfoods is the omega-3

long-chain unsaturated fats EPA and DHA. For a considerable length of time omega-3s have been the esteemed most loved of the nutritional wellbeing world. What we didn't know already, which we do now, is that they additionally improve the action of a subset of sirtuin qualities in the body that are straightforwardly connected to life span. This makes them the ideal blending with Sirtfoods.

Omega-3s have intense impacts in lessening inflammation and decreasing the degree of fats in the blood. To that we can include extra heart-healthy impacts: they make the blood more averse to cluster, balance out the electrical cadence of the heart, and cut down pulse. Indeed, even the pharmaceutical business is currently going to them as a guide in the fight against coronary illness. What's more, the reiteration of advantages doesn't end there. Omega-3s additionally influence the manner in which we think, having been appeared to improve mind-set just as assisting with fighting off dementia.

At the point when we talk about omega-3s we're basically looking at eating fish, explicitly the sleek assortments, on the grounds that no other dietary source verges on giving the critical degrees of EPA and DHA we need. And all we need so as to see the advantages is two servings of fish seven days, with an accentuation on sleek sh. sadly, the US isn't a country of huge fish eaters, and less than one out of five Americans accomplish this. Subsequently, our admission of the valuable EPA and DHA comes up woefully short.

Plant nourishments, for example, nuts, seeds, and green verdant vegetables additionally contain omega-3 however in a structure called alpha-linoleic corrosive, which should be changed over to EPA or DHA in the body. This transformation procedure is poor, which implies that alpha-linoleic corrosive gives an immaterial measure of our omega-3 needs. Indeed, even with the awesome advantages from Sirtfoods, we ought not to ignore the additional worth those devouring adequate degrees of omega-3 fats bring.

The best omega-3 fish sources are herring, sardines, salmon, trout, and mackerel, in a specific order. While new fish is normally high as well, most of the omega-3 is lost in the tinned form. Furthermore, for veggie lovers and vegetarians, while plant sources should in any case be fused into the diet, an enhancement of DHA-advanced microalgae (up to 300 milligrams per day) is likewise energized.

Just as being a significant omega-3 and protein source, slick fish is a phenomenal wellspring of nutrients and minerals, for example, nutrients An and D, B nutrients, and follow minerals including iodine and zinc. The suggestion for grown-ups is to eat in any event two servings of fish, of which one is slick fish, seven days.

CAN A SIRTFOOD DIET GIVE EVERYTHING?

So far our spotlight has been exclusively on Sirtfoods and receiving their most extreme rewards with the goal that we can accomplish the body we need and effectively support our wellbeing all the while. Be that as it may, is this a dependable dietary way to deal with be taking as long as possible? All things considered, there is a whole other world to diet than just sirtuin-enacting supplements.

Shouldn't something be said about all the nutrients, minerals, and fiber that are likewise fundamental for our prosperity and the nourishments we ought to eat to fulfill those requests? Intriguingly, what we find is that when we maintain a solid spotlight on Sirtfoods, supplemented by protein-rich nourishments and wellsprings of omega-3, dietary needs are fulfilled over the entire range of fundamental supplements—substantially more so than by some other diet, truth be told.

For instance, we incorporate kale since it is a powerful Sirtfood, yet it is additionally an incredible wellspring of nutrients C and K, foliate, and the minerals manganese, calcium, and magnesium. Just as resistant boosting beta-carotene, kale is likewise a gigantic wellspring of the carotenoids lutein and zeaxanthin, the two of which are basic in eye wellbeing.

Moreover, pecans are plentiful in minerals including magnesium, copper, zinc, manganese, calcium, and iron, just as fiber. Buckwheat is brimming with manganese, copper, magnesium, potassium, and fiber. Onions mark the containers for nutrient B6, foliate, potassium, and fiber. Furthermore, strawberries are great wellsprings of nutrient C just as potassium and manganese. Thus it goes on. When you expand your diet to incorporate the all-inclusive Sirtfood list, just as saving space for each one of those other great nourishments you appreciate eating; accidentally what you will really wind up with is a diet far more extravagant in nutrients, minerals, and fiber than you at any point had previously. As a result, what Sirtfoods offer is a missing nutrition type that changes the scene of how we judge how great nourishments are for us, and how we eat a genuinely complete diet.

BALANCING PLANT-BASED DIETS

Sirtfoods are a festival of the best plant nourishments on earth. So it should not shock anyone those veggie lovers, who normally remember a greater amount of them for their diet, have been appeared to have lower paces of malignant growth, diabetes, coronary illness, and corpulence. Specialists, for example, the renowned Foundation of Nutrition and Dietetics are vociferous in their help of vegan diets, expressing that they are refreshing and nutritionally satisfactory, and may give medical advantages in the counteraction and treatment of specific ailments. Plant-based cooking is deserving of its own applauses and meriting a spot on anybody's supper table. As of now you will have encountered this for yourself, with the consideration of dishes, for example, the Butternut Squash and Date Tagine with Buckwheat in Stage 2 for vegans and carnivores the same, offering plant-based admission at its best. In any case, with regards to eating exclusively plant-based vegetarian diets, it's an alternate issue. Tantamount to Sirtfoods are, the diet can miss the mark. Without creature protein to supplement Sirtfoods, there is a danger of nutritional insufficiencies.

We've just perceived how fundamental omega-3 unsaturated fats are for wellbeing and how plant sources are deficient. Along these lines our proposal for veggie lovers and vegetarians is for a

DHA- advanced microalgae supplement to be taken day by day.

Veggie lovers and particularly vegetarians can likewise end up lacking nutrient B12. We can just get nutrient B12 from creature items (counting dairy and eggs), so eat only plant nourishments and sometime you'll end up insufficient. In the event that we become insufficient in nutrient B12, we put ourselves at expanded danger of coronary illness, sickliness, neurological degeneration, wretchedness, and dementia. On the off chance that you wish to eat a carefully plant-based diet, the most ideal route around this problem is to take nutrient B12 as an enhancement.

Calcium is another key supplement vegetarians should know about: there is a 30 percent more prominent rate of breaks in veggie lovers because of low calcium admission. While it is conceivable to get calcium from a plant-based diet, you have to put forth a cognizant attempt. Great plant wellsprings of calcium incorporate green vegetables (e.g., kale, broccoli), calcium-strengthened refreshments (soy milk, almond milk, and rice milk), and tofu set with calcium, nuts, and seeds. All things being equal, a moderate calcium supplement might be required.

At last, exceptionally high paces of iodine lack (80 percent in veggie lovers and 25 percent in vegans) have been found in individuals eating exclusively plant-based diets. Iodine is imperative for making thyroid hormones, which are totally basic in managing digestion. With dietary sources being fish, fish, and milk, veggie lovers run into inconvenience. Luckily, devouring iodized salt is a powerful method for boosting your iodine levels, and it is generally accessible in supermarkets. However, for veggie lovers not utilizing a calculable measure of iodized salt, an enhancement is likely required.

While kelp is an exceptionally rich wellspring of iodine, it can contain very high and possibly over the top levels, which is similarly as awful for the thyroid as getting close to nothing, and ought not to be depended upon.

THE PHYSICAL MOVEMENT IMPACT

The Sirtfood Diet is tied in with eating those nourishments structured ordinarily to advance supported weight loss and prosperity. Yet, with the advantages you see from following the diet, it is conceivable to fall into the snare of feeling that there is no compelling reason to work out. Many diet books will embrace this, saying how incapable exercise is contrasted with following the right diet for weight loss. Furthermore, it's actual; we can't out-practice a terrible diet. As we saw before, it's not the way that was planned to drive weight loss. It's wasteful, and a lot of fringes on being hurtful. So the facts confirm that there's no compelling reason to pound the treadmill until we are seeing stars or play out the accomplishments of an Olympian—yet shouldn't something be said about general ordinary development?

The truth of the matter is we are far less dynamic now than we used to be. The time of innovation, for all the advances it has brought, has implied physical action is practically calculated out of our everyday lives. Except if we really need to, we truly don't need to waste time with the entire business of being dynamic. We can turn up, drive to work, take the lift, sit at a work area throughout the day, commute home, eat, and sit in front of the television before folding into bed once more, at that point do the equivalent the following day, and the following.

Disregard weight loss for a second and simply investigate the reiteration of medical advantages being dynamic is connected to. These incorporate decreased danger of cardiovascular ailment, stroke, hypertension, type 2 diabetes, osteoporosis, weight, and malignant growth just as improved disposition, rest, condense, and feeling of prosperity. While great deals of the advantages of being dynamic are passed through turning on our sirtuin qualities, we ought not to utilize eating Sirtfoods as an explanation not to take part in work out. Or maybe we ought to acknowledge how being dynamic is the ideal supplement to our utilization of Sirtfoods. This invigorates most extreme sirtuin actuation, and all the advantages that brings, precisely as nature proposed.

What we are discussing here is meeting government rules of 150 minutes (2 hours and 30 minutes) of moderate physical movement seven days.

Moderate movement is what might be compared to an energetic walk. In any case, it doesn't need to be limited to this. Any game or physical action you appreciate is appropriate. Delight and exercise don't should be fundamentally unrelated! What's more, group or network sports are enhanced even more by their social viewpoint. It's about everyday things as well, such as taking the bicycle rather than the vehicle, or getting off the transport one stop prior, or just leaving more distant away to expand the separation you need to walk. Use the stairwell rather than the lift. Head outside and do some planting. Play with your children in the recreation center, or get out additional with the canine. Everything checks. Performed normally, and at moderate force, whatever has you up and moving will enact your sirtuin qualities, upgrading the advantages of the Sirtfood Diet.

Taking part in physical action while eating a Sirtfood-rich diet gives most extreme sirtuin value for your money. All that is expected to accomplish the physical movement impact is what might be compared to an energetic 30-minute walk five times each week.

RUNDOWN

- While the best twenty Sirtfoods ought to stay in the focal point of the plate, there are numerous different plants with sirtuin-initiating properties that ought to be remembered for our diets to make them changed and various.

- A diet rich in Sirtfoods supplemented by the incorporation of creature items and fish gives all the advantages of sirtuin initiation, just as addressing the requirement for other basic supplements.

- While veggie lovers and vegans can get all the advantages from a Sirtfood-based diet, cautious consideration ought to be given to those supplements that might be missing and proper food decisions or supplementation made. Supporters of the Sirtfood Diet are urged to participate in moderate movement for thirty minutes five times each week to receive the numerous rewards of activity for prosperity and animate most extreme sirtuin enactment.

CHAPTER TWELVE:
SIRTFOODS FOR ALL

As we traveled further and more profound into the magnificent universe of Sirtfoods, we started to acknowledge exactly how wide their application could be. We're extremely mindful that no two individuals eat the equivalent, and numerous wellbeing cognizant individuals are firmly dedicated to a specific method of eating, with any semblance of paleo, low carb, discontinuous fasting, and without gluten diets being particularly mainstream. While they don't work for a few, others depend on them. In any case, exactly how do Sirtfoods t in with these?

A light second hit with the acknowledgment that each and every one of these well-known diets would be incredibly upgraded if Sirtfoods were coordinated into them. The advantages individuals were getting from them—wellbeing or weight loss— could be enhanced just through the expansion of Sirtfoods in adequate amounts. Along these lines, Sirtfoods are all inclusive: if there's a method of eating that truly works for you, fusing Sirtfoods into it will make your outcomes shockingly better.

We're both occupied clinicians, and as our excitement for Sirtfoods has developed, we have incorporated Sirtfoods increasingly more unequivocally into the diets of the customers we work with, regardless of what their favored method of eating. Our decision is clear: not exclusively are Sirtfoods perfect with all other dietary methodologies, they intensely upgrade them. Truth be told, they ought to be fundamental fixings in each mainstream diet. Ignore them and you're truly missing a stunt.

PALEO DIET

More or less, the paleo diet advances that we ought to eat the nourishments that it is assumed our old precursors were eating, before the coming of present day horticulture and all the more as of late modern food handling. Basically we're talking a tracker gatherer or Stone Age man style of diet, comprising of meats, fish and shell fish, vegetables, organic products, and nuts, while banished to the wild are dairy items, oat grains, sugar, and every handled food.

For paleo dieters, we suggest this conversation starter: what could be more paleo than eating the plant nourishments with which we've coevolved that switch on our antiquated sirtuin qualities? You will review that the two plants and creatures have created methods of adapting to normal ecological anxieties, for example, parchedness, sun introduction, absence of supplements, and assault by aggressors.

On account of their inactive nature (they can't flee!), plants have grown particularly refined pressure reaction frameworks, creating a mind boggling cluster of polyphenols that permit them to adapt to their condition. For centuries, people have been ingesting these polyphenols, piggybacking on these complex pressure reaction signals created by plants and receiving enormous rewards as they switch all alone sirtuin qualities.

What could be more paleo than devouring the sirtuin-initiating plant aggravates our tracker gatherer progenitors would have blossomed with? Sirtfoods are the missing bit of the paleo theory.

LOW-CARB DIET

Since the time Atkins, the dad of low-carb diets, rose to transient reputation, lowcarb diets have been a significant milestone on the weight-loss map. Resulting resurrections, for example, the Dukan diet, have kept on energizing the low-carb development. Among them, they have indented diet-book deals up to the several millions. While such low-carb diets can be extraordinary, particularly in their initial "ambush" stages, their wide assessments do mirror a more extensive move in conclusion toward an enemy of sugar and even enemy of carb position. Progressively individuals are deserting the sinking boat of the low-fat worldview and moving loyalties to the "carbs are the foe" camp.

One of the wonders of the Sirtfood Diet is that it doesn't include this regional clash. It's a diet of consideration, which implies that you truly don't need to pick sides and bar an entire nutrition class from your diet so as to accomplish the body you need. By and by, we value that numerous individuals have an inclination for a lower-carb style of eating, so where do Sirtfoods t in?

On the off chance that your influence is toward low-carb, at that point we encourage you not to ration Sirtfoods, however to grasp them. We would say, perhaps the greatest snare we see individuals fall into when eating low-carb diets is the absence of plant based nourishments they contain. Suppers become vigorously situated around meats (and frequently handled meats); fish, eggs, cheddar, and other dairy items, and plant based nourishments get consigned to the base of the hierarchy.

Yet, on the off chance that it's low carb, it's all acceptable . . . or on the other hand so we're told. Too bad, the thought those plant-based nourishments aren't of focal significance in our diets goes against practically all that we think about diet and wellbeing. A diet exhausted of the huge swath of helpful mixes found in plant nourishments will do little to turn away a torrential slide of interminable ailments, for example, dementia, coronary illness, and malignancy.

However it is completely conceivable to incorporate a wealth of Sirtfoods into a carb-confined method of eating. Simply take a gander at the main twenty arrangements of Sirtfoods and you will find that a lion's shares of them are naturally low in carbs. We're discussing an abundance of verdant and low-carb vegetables (arugula, celery, endive, kale, and onions), culinary herbs (garlic, parsley), flavors (bean stew, turmeric), tricks, pecans, cocoa, and additional virgin olive oil, not overlooking the drinks (espresso and green tea). Concerning natural product, so frequently the objective of assault on low-carb diets, even the strawberries say something with a negligible teaspoon of sugars from a liberal 3 1/2-ounce (100g) serving.

For us the reality is this: no low-carb diet ought to be a low-

Sirtfood diet. Not exclusively does consolidating Sirtfoods upgrade the weight-loss advantages of a low-carb diet, however it significantly builds its wellbeing potential.

IRREGULAR FASTING/THE 5:2 DIET

Irregular fasting, otherwise called IF, has become an enormous dietary marvel over the most recent couple of years, encapsulated by the runaway accomplishment of the 5:2 diets. This commonly includes limiting calorie admission to 500 to 600 calories for each day on two days out of every week, and eating anything you desire on the other five days.

While strong investigation into the advantages of discontinuous fasting is still entirely constrained, it appears to be valuable for weight loss and improving a portion of the hazard factors for ailment. Be that as it may, as we've seen, it's not appropriate for huge sections of the populace, it causes unfortunate muscle loss, and it's just powerful in the event that you can adhere to it. What's more, that truly is the glaring issue at hand with regards to irregular fasting and why we're not excessively captivated with it. As far as we can tell, most of individuals neglect to adhere to irregular fasting regimens for any obvious period of time. Yearning is an unsavory inclination that chews away at you, so obviously individuals simply don't care to feel hungry that regularly.

While irregular fasting has not ended up being a panacea, it is well known for an explanation, and there will be fans that depend on its advantages. We completely regard this, obviously. Be that as it may, why not give your quick a genuine updating by "Sirtifying" it?

With the presentation of Sirtfoods, you will get all the advantages they bring to lessen the unfavorable impacts of fasting, including assisting with satisfying appetite and protect muscle. In any case, there's another enormous reward to their incorporation. You will recollect that the advantages of fasting are interceded through the initiation of our sirtuin qualities, which is additionally precisely how Sirtfoods work. This implies with Sirtfoods now present to share the fasting "trouble," you can up your calorie admission to a substantially more reasonable level while as yet receiving no different rewards.

This is actually what we have found in our clinical practice. With simply the consideration of Sirtfood- rich green squeezes (a similar formula utilized in this book) in a typical IF menu, supporters have had the option to expand their vitality admission from a serious 500 to 600 calories on quick days to a substantially more reasonable 800 to 1,000 calories.

So if your propensity is for discontinuous fasting, you're feeling the loss of a stunt and making quick days unduly difficult by not grasping Sirtfoods. Truth be told, there's an entire other point from which discontinuous fasting diets would profit by grasping Sirtfoods. With IF diets there are practically nothing, assuming any, attention on the nature of the food; it's everything about the calorie deficit on quick days. Truth be told, defenders are vociferous in supporting that you can eat anything you desire on non-quick days.

Regardless of whether what you eat is acceptable, awful, or inside and out awful doesn't generally appear to issue. Be that as it may, as we probably are aware, the body needs a ceaseless flexibly of fundamental supplements to keep everything working fit as a fiddle. Will we truly hope to pull off denying the assortment of basic nutrition by eating whatever supplement stripped, prepared nourishments we need, regardless of whether we are fasting for two days, and fight off interminable ailments like Alzheimer's or coronary illness?

Consider the possibility that, then again, you likewise included supplement thick Sirtfoods on your non-fasting days. You would never again be consuming fat and upgrading wellbeing only two days per week—it would now be seven. To us this advancement of the irregular fasting approach is an easy decision. It's what could be compared to updating a high contrast television to full-shading HD. Sans gluten DIET

The excellence of the Sirtfood Diet for any individual who needs to keep away from gluten is that the main twenty Sirtfoods are all normally without gluten. Gluten is a kind of protein found in wheat, rye, and grain. A few people with gluten prejudice can likewise be delicate to oats (through cross- sullying). Victims of the immune system issue celiac malady, which influences upwards of 1 of every 100 individuals in America, are easily affected to gluten and can't devour it in any structure, however beside this intense gluten narrow mindedness, numerous individuals are progressively trying different things with without gluten diets and regularly discover they feel better on them.

At the point when individuals set out on without gluten diets, which include removing staples, for example, bread, pasta, and the bunch of different nourishments produced using gluten containing grains, one of the huge concerns is that the diet turns out to be nutritionally inadequate and no longer gives the full scope of supplements and fiber expected to remain healthy. What's so extraordinary about the Sirtfood Diet is that one of our top Sirtfoods is buckwheat, a normally sans gluten and profoundly nutritious pseudo-grain, which, as we have seen through the former sections, is adaptable enough to step in as a swap for gluten-containing grains, regardless of whether as our, pasta, pieces, or noodles (check the bundle cautiously to guarantee that these are 100 percent buckwheat).

Obviously, the best diets are the ones that are assorted and changed, not redundant and dreary. We saw that quinoa, another pseudo-grain, are without gluten as well as have important measures of sirtuin-actuating supplements, making it the ideal reinforcement to buckwheat.

Beside its standard pretense as a grain, quinoa is progressively accessible as our, chips, and pasta from wellbeing food stores and claims to fame online providers. With quinoa and buckwheat becoming the dominant focal point, it's upbeat days for anybody receiving a sans gluten diet: in addition to the fact that they offer an advantageous option in contrast to different grains, yet including them as staple nourishments adds some genuine

Sirtfood certifications to the normal diet. We can't leave the subject of sans gluten diets without an expression of caution about the mass of sans gluten low quality nourishment that currently tops off the "free from" racks in each market.

These are the profoundly handled, refined, sweet, without gluten options in contrast to cakes, bread rolls, treats, breakfast oats, etc. This has become an enormous industry; however kindly don't fall into the snare of reasoning that on the grounds that an item is without gluten it is essentially healthy. Most of these nourishments are nutritionally unfilled garbage, much the same as their gluten-containing partners. On the off chance that you are following a without gluten diet, we ask you to all up on a tight eating routine rich in normally sans gluten Sirtfoods, not sans gluten garbage, and take your wellbeing and prosperity to an unheard of level.

OUTLINE

- Sirtfoods are good with all other dietary methodologies as well as effectively upgrade their advantages.
- Sirtfoods are the model paleo nourishments, containing the sirtuin-enacting polyphenols that people have developed eating, and receiving the rewards from, over innumerable centuries.
- Low-carb diets that need plant-based nourishments can be drastically improved by the incorporation of Sirtfoods.
- Eating a diet rich in Sirtfoods implies that the calorie limitation of discontinuous fasting can be less extreme, yet the advantages will be the equivalent if not more noteworthy.

The best twenty Sirtfoods are normally sans gluten, making them a help for anybody following a sans gluten diet.

CHAPTER THIRTEEN: SOCIAL EFFECTS ON OBESITY IN SIRTFOOD DIET

Youth and pre-grown-up heftiness have an arrangement of causes. Among them are genetic characteristics; earlier weight status; and family, peer, and social effects. The objective of this part is to plot the effects of family, peer, and social consequences for the physiological and social choices made by preadolescents and adolescents that may fabricate their threat of getting overweight or fat. We study composing on modifiable determinants of heftiness and weight gain.

Disregarding the way that affiliations developed in clinical fundamentals have been exhibited to be less disposed to confusing and decision tendency than observational examinations, clinical primers don't helpfully credit themselves to the appraisal of family, peer, and social effects. We place increasingly imperative burden on longitudinal assessments among the observational examinations since common solicitation of affiliations can be set up.

FAMILIAL EFFECTS

Watchmen sway their youths' weight through the two characteristics and practices. One trial of looking at familial effects is unwinding the activity of characteristics from the activity of natural factors. Also, it is attempting to detach determinants of common and sound weight gain from those related to excessive weight gain since adolescents and young people are depended upon to create and gain weight during a ton of youth and youthfulness. This may be one explanation that couples of direct factors have been dependably perceived in observational assessments as pointers of over the top weight expansion or corpulence during youth and youthfulness.

BEGINNING TIMES AND YOUTH

Various developmental changes occur during the underlying 18 years of life. In youth, gatekeepers tremendously affect what their adolescent eats and, subsequently, on the child's risk of putting on an extreme proportion of weight. In any case, as children age and contribute more vitality away from home at school, in day care, and in after school programs, parental effect begins to vanish. Posterity of overweight mothers has been viewed as more likely than their slenderer allies to get overweight.

This connection likely reflects both inherited and social effects. Whitaker thought low-pay children and saw that when mothers were hefty in early pregnancy their adolescents were more than twice as inclined to be enormous at 2 to 4 years of age.

In addition, a couple of assessments have found that adolescents bound to women who were once previously (i.e., pre-pregnancy) overweight will undoubtedly be overweight as well. Overweight and hefty mothers have all the reserves of being more amazing than their less greasy companions to chest feed their adolescents. This lead choice may furthermore grow the infant kid's threat of getting overweight. Liberated from the mother's weight, a couple of assessments have seen that the more expanded an infant youngster is just chest dealt with (or gets chest milk just), the lower the child's risk is of getting overweight later in youth or adolescence.

In any case, the connection has not been found in a couple of various examinations. Some anomaly in the disclosures may have come about as a result of changing model size, length of improvement, and implications of chest dealing with exposures (i.e., any chest dealing with, just chest dealing with and not upgrading with condition or solids, and range of chest dealing with). Dealing with practices of watchmen other than chest dealing with similarly sway the weight status and weight expansion of their infants and little children. Deplorably, the amount of longitudinal examinations that have studied the directionality of a youth's weight status and the dealing with practices of their people is obliged.

Posterity of mothers with high stresses over their infant youngster glutting or ending up being overweight gotten on a very basic level more muscle versus fat over 2 years than did their companions whose mothers were not as concerned. It is obfuscated how mothers' inclinations changed over into real dealing with rehearses, anyway constraint of explicit sustenance's or sorts of sustenance's may have been one lead included. Fisher and Birch found that increasingly raised degrees of maternal restriction to sustenance get to where related with progressively important snack sustenance utilization among their 3-to 5-year-old young ladies.

What's more, higher maternal sustenance impediment was connected with the mother's own dietary restriction similarly likewise with raised degrees of muscle versus fat among their youths. Also, Certainty et al found that parental impediment foreseen weight list (BMI) increases in adolescents over a 2-year time span (from ages 5 to 7). These results suggest that although a segment of the maternal constraint may be amiable (i.e., to thwart superfluous weight gain among kids with high muscle to fat proportion), restriction may invert release and be connected with increasingly critical admission of limited sustenance's when the child is offered access to them.

In a review of finds out about parental restrictive dealing with style, Certainty and Kerns found that in numerous examinations, youth qualities, for instance, being overweight, were related to restrictive dealing with points of view and styles of their people. Taken together, the results suggest that mothers of overweight children will undoubtedly be stressed over their adolescent's weight and may try to constrain the child's sustenance admission. Continuously up and coming examination is relied upon to all the more promptly appreciate whether maternal impediment is profitable or negative.

Maternal weight concerns and constraints may affect more than a child's weight status; they may in like manner sway their certainty and feelings about their weight. Research suggests that adolescents as young as 5 years may be conversely affected by their mother's tension about their weight. In the National Turn of events and Prosperity Study saw that around 40% of High differentiation youngsters who were 9 or 10 years old were endeavoring to get more slender. High BMI and having a mother unveil to her daughter she was too fat were connected with consistent keeping away from over the top food consumption among the youngsters. Tragically, given the cross-sectional arrangement of the assessment, it is obfuscated whether the youngsters were extremely overweight or whether the young ladies' weight decrease tries were convincing. In a tinier longitudinal assessment, Francis and Birch followed and reviewed 173 mothers and their young ladies at 5, 7, 9, and 11 years of age.

They found that mothers fascinated with their own weight and eating uncovered progressively huge degrees of keeping their young ladies' admission and enabling weight decrease in their daughters.

Additionally, maternal reassurance of weight decrease was unequivocally related to young ladies' controlled eating conduct.

Although pediatric heftiness is a colossal general clinical issue, and thusly reveling should be discouraged, controlled eating may progress rather than prevent weight gain. A couple of longitudinal assessments have seen that inconceivably, liberated from standard BMI, eating less lousy nourishment is connected with gaining more weight; along these lines, familial components that advance going without exorbitant food admission or impediment may subsequently propel progressively vital weight gain.

PREADOLESCENCE AND ADOLESCENCE

The hour of preadolescence and adolescence may be particularly noteworthy in the expectation of overweight and weight. The normality of pre-grown-up overweight has extended practically triple since the late 1980s, and weight status during preadolescence and pubescence is an average pointer of adult weight status.

As children become preadolescents and subsequently youngsters, they become progressively independent and choose their own special more prominent sum choices. Through this season of headway, gatekeepers have continuously less order over what their youths eat considering the way that young people right presently may be purchasing greater sustenance outside of the home, including modest food, sugar-improved beverages, and other convenience food sources with high caloric substance and regardless broken healthy advantage that may improve the likelihood of preposterous weight gain.

Youth's right presently moreover may finish up whether to partake in sports and when and where they have to eat and drink. Additionally, they may end up being dynamically mindful of their weight and thusly get practices to change their weight or shape. Not under any condition like little children who may need to grasp the practices that will fulfill their people, a couple of youngsters may be progressively excited about getting rehearses that their companions will support of and have less energy for complying with their people's proposals.

Albeit parental effects are up 'til now critical at this age, particularly for preadolescents and youngsters living at home, social weights, the obvious feelings and lead of their buddies, media pictures, and displaying sway direct in any occasion as much as do watchmen.

EATING BEHAVIOR

Since watchmen are more likely than their children to buy and prepare sustenance, they accept a key activity in propelling sound or terrible dietary models by showing eating plans and offering access to nutritious sustenance's at home. Various gatekeepers inadvertently send conflicting messages about food. Parental admission was a tremendous pointer of dairy, natural item, and vegetable admission. Strangely, verdant nourishments admission was immaterial to the youngsters' admissions. More research is required to grasp the sex differentiation in the effect of parental showing of sound dietary practices. Albeit parental exhibiting of eating nourishments developed starting from the earliest stage not assessed, in an examination of 3,957 youngsters in Minnesota.

Regardless, if availability was high, even young people who couldn't have cared less for the taste ate up a greater number of nourishments developed starting from the earliest stage their colleagues in homes with low openness. In a resulting report, saw that parental admission while the individuals were youngster's basically foreseen admission of normal items, vegetables, and dairy sustenance's 5 years sometime later.

Taken together, the results suggest that openness of nourishments developed starting from the earliest stage crucial, anyway further research is relied upon to choose the relationship of parental showing of dietary practices and the following dietary demonstrations of their youths. Amazingly, various fiscally troubled systems have very few gigantic general stores.

In such cases, verdant nourishments may be out of reach or preposterously expensive for watchmen and parental figures to purchase in sufficient sums. Watchmen can in like manner sway their children's eating structures by having the family eat suppers together. A variety of points of interest has been connected with eating meals with family, for instance, expectation of superfluous weight gains and less pre-grown-up use of tobacco, alcohol, and cannabis in a cross-sectional examination of 7,784 youngsters and 6,647 youngsters developed 9 to 14 years in the Growing Up Today Study (GUTS), an imminent partner assessment, Gillman et al saw that preadolescents had dinner more as frequently as conceivable with their family than did young people.

For the most part, 17% of individuals only sometimes ate with their family, 40% ate with them on most days, and 43% ate with relative's step by step. Free mature enough and sexual direction, youths who a significant part of the time ate with their family were will undoubtedly eat at any rate five servings of verdant food sources each day and were out and out progressively loath to drink pop or obliterate any burned sustenance's from home. Among 4,746 youngsters in Adventure EAT found that repeat of family dinners was decidedly associated with admission of nourishments developed starting from the earliest stage conflictingly associated with soft drink usage. Folks, focus school understudies, youngsters whose mothers didn't work, and adolescents with higher money related status (SES), were will undoubtedly consume family dinners.

The association between family meals and high suggests that it is possible that family dinners are one framework through which high-SES individuals decay their threat of getting overweight or large. On the other hand, it is possible that eating family meals together may appear, apparently, to be connected with acceptable dieting plans since it is a middle person for high SES.

The limitation of cross-sectional assessments is that one can't choose directionality of affiliations or explore frameworks. The longitudinal data on eating family suppers and coming about weight change are obliged and dubious. In the GUTS assistant, saw that despite the way that at standard the more as regularly as conceivable an adolescent ate with their family the more abnormal the individual was to be overweight, the repeat of eating family suppers didn't predict whether the child got overweight during the following year. One potential explanation for the nonattendance of longitudinal association could be that kids who are outstandingly unique, which would be protective against the progression of weight, may play on sports bunches that preparation or have games now and again that intrude with eating with their family.

Mixing these adolescents in with kids who don't eat with their family for less strong reasons would debilitate any relationship of a protective effect of family dinner. Another possible explanation is that not all family dinners are strong or have fitting piece sizes. Heftiness is referred to gather in families because of a mix of inherited and environmental effects; along these lines, it is possible that family dinner in families with overweight or enormous gatekeepers may be depicted by pointless calories and in this way don't guarantee against excessive weight gain.

WEIGHT CONCERNS AND WEIGHT CONTROL PRACTICES

Watchmen should think about their own weight-related attitudes and weight control rehearses similarly as their points of view toward their youth's weight to keep up a key good ways from surprising progression of body frustration and weight stresses among their children. In GUTS, Field et al found that youths' acknowledgment that their weight was basic to their father was connected with getting stressed over their weight paying little regard to their real BMI.

Furthermore, both Field saw that preadolescents' and adolescents' perspective on their mother's weight control practices and weight concerns were connected with the youth's own weight concerns and weight control rehearses. In addition, Field found that self-ruling of an adolescent's or young BMI, the people who diet put on more weight than their companions. These results recommend that family of watchmen with weight concerns may be at progressively genuine danger for weight gain by showing their practices on the impression of the gatekeepers' practices and feelings. Partner Effects Notwithstanding the way that friends sway kids at all ages, peer sway is more vital during preadolescence and energy than youth. During preadolescence and youth, affirmation by peers is significantly regarded, and to get this affirmation, youngsters may grasp the clear feelings and practices practiced by people from their companion gathering.

The aching to be charming to companions can affect decisions about participating in sound similarly as shocking practices. Among preadolescent and juvenile youngsters, progressively vital criticalness is determined to body weight and shape among heteros than lesbians. As youngsters enter pubescence, they may get deplorable weight control rehearses, for instance, skipping breakfast or using diet pills or intestinal meds to control their weight. Furthermore, ending up being pulled in to youngsters may cause post pubertal young women who have made androgen-related changes (e.g., individual odor, pubic hair) to end up being less arranged to look into practices that they acknowledge may make them really terrible?

This avoidance could make them especially exposed against putting on irrational proportions of weight considering the way that their imperativeness use would be reducing while the hormonal changes of youthfulness are beginning, causing additions by and large fat mass. Companion impacts on lifestyle practices can be negative; anyway a couple of assessments have researched whether peer-based participation and social weight can be used to determinedly impact prosperity and risk direct. Since particular characteristics may change as per peer-pack guidelines and characteristics, sidekicks may expect a noteworthy activity in choosing eating routine and activity instances of adolescents and young people.

Unfortunately, only two or three investigations have assessed peer consequences for diet and development plans that may affect the threat of heftiness. A couple of interventions have used a sort of buddy genuine guides to propel a strong eating schedule. In the Young people Eating for Essentialness and Food at School intervention, which had a school area mediations arm, a homeroom notwithstanding class condition mediations arm, and a buddy boss notwithstanding an investigation lobby and school condition mediations arm, it was found that kids in the companion heads notwithstanding study corridor and school condition interventions arm made the greatest constructive changes in dietary admission.

These results prescribe that interventions to propel strong dietary models would be sagacious to incorporate companions as genuine models and promoters of the intercession. Social norms may be a huge and understudied determinant of lifestyle related to weight evasion. A creating array of composing recommends that social gauges sway keeping away from extreme food admission and tragic weight control practices of adolescents. The activity of companion sway in the lessening in physical development as youngster's headway through preadolescence and youthfulness is less thought of. In any case, as youngsters progress through youth to preadolescence and youthfulness, they will when all is said in done turn out to be progressively aware of their appearance and may end up being less arranged to check out activities that could impact their haircuts, make-up, or nails. These concerns have not been packed in emotional or quantitative examinations yet have been represented to the makers of this part by physical guidance teachers, so it is obfuscated how ordinary these concerns are and what influence they have on the decline in physical activity among youngsters. Not all companion impacts are on a very basic level negative, regardless. Partners may similarly propel sound practices. Among 354 youngsters who were 8 to 11 years of age, those whose friends and family maintained practice were practically sure than their allies to make part in physical move.

These results prescribe that to viably propel activity and thwart corpulence among female youth, it may be sensible to advance endeavors to change peer gauges to help and worth being dynamic and eating a strong eating routine. Regardless, significantly more research is required to all the almost certain appreciate the relationship of partner guidelines and impacts on diet and activity instances of preadolescent and energetic youngsters.

SOCIAL EFFECTS

Huge impacts on kids, other than those of loved ones, are the school condition and media. Schools offer opportunities to adolescents to both purchase and eat up sustenance, and they are also in a circumstance to affect eating practices and activity levels through investigation corridor and sports programs. Outside of school, youths contribute a ton of vitality gazing at the television, which opens them to publicizing for normally unwanted sustenance things.

This portion looks at these segments and the frameworks by which they may extend the peril of weight among children and youngsters.

CHAPTER FOURTEEN:
PSYCHOSOCIAL OUTCOMES OF OBESITY
AND WEIGHT IN SIRTFOOD

Obesity is connected with hostile physical and mental results. Regardless of the way that the physical results are a quick delayed consequence of obesity, the psychological results are primarily an outcome of weight tendency. Interventions are necessitated that intend to hinder juvenile and youth obesity similarly as decay the various sorts of weight-related maligning that occur in our overall population. To help in the progression of such mediations, a dear understanding of the relationship among obesity, weight-related criticism, and hostile psychosocial results is moreover required.

Our assessment bunch has focused on endeavoring to all the almost certain appreciate the experience of being overweight in a slim organized society. A ton of our work has attempted to manufacture our cognizance of the psychosocial results of obesity and weight tendency to control the improvement of interventions got ready for preventing obesity and other weight-related messes among children and youngsters. For example, we have examined the repeat and impact of weight- related goading in children and youngsters to choose the size of the issue, whether or not it is meriting tending to inside interventions, and how best to address weight-pushing to decrease its occasion.

We have used quantitative, emotional, and intervention ask about strategies to explore weight- related analysis, psychosocial concerns, and prosperity dealing rehearses among 79 overweight youth. Quantitative investigations of tremendous masses based models have been useful in taking a gander at relationship among weight and its psychosocial results. Start to finish gatherings and focus social events with humbler instances of youths and young people have given additional information about their experiences overseeing weight-based trashing. Our intervention investigate with adolescents and young people has taught us about issues, for instance, self-discernment concerns and weight goading, domains that we are reliably endeavoring to address even more effectively through work with youth similarly likewise with their educators, guides, youth pack pioneers, social protection providers, and gatekeepers.

At the present time, take a gander at the psychosocial consequences of obesity and weight tendency recognized in our own assessment and in made by others. We first present a segment of the key research revelations taking a gander at the social results of being overweight inside an overall population that characteristics slimness. We by then glance at the implications of being overweight and of being introduced to weight-related mocking on mental thriving and discussion about recommendations for moving toward the shirking of obesity, weight tendency, and their related psychosocial results.

CRITICISM AND MALTREATMENT BY COMPANIONS

Weight is conflictingly generalized in Western social orders, and this negative generalizing appears to begin directly off the bat for the duration of regular day to day existence. Studies have found that kids as energetic as 3 years' characteristic negative characteristics, for instance, "detached," "messy," "stupid," "revolting," "liar," and "cheat," to overweight children. In a movement of achievement inspects drove in the mid-1960s, 10- and 11-year-old children were shown six drawings of children and were drawn nearer to rank them according to how well they appreciated each child. The drawings consolidated a sound adolescent, an obesity child, and four children with various physical debilitations or distortions. The youths situated the obesity kid prop up on amiability, behind the children with physical deterrents including facial misshaping and use of a wheelchair. It is indistinguishable how these theoretical circumstances reflect the certified experiences of enormous youth.

One assessment has suggested that points of view may be progressively positive, taking everything into account, conditions than in these undeniably special conditions;

Lawson found no association between the speculations joined to drawings and same-thing choices of overweight companions among a case of 84 youths in Assessments 2 through 6. In like manner, the charming gauges relating to body shape didn't have all the reserves of being used to evaluate their individual partners. Correspondingly, Phillips and Incline found that overweight preadolescent youngsters got peer assignments of reputation like those of common weight young women. Then again, as delineated in the going with areas, different examinations have found that overweight youth are needy upon various sorts of maltreatment by their sidekicks, including social detachment or minimization, weight-related pushing, and bothering.

ANALYSIS AND MALTREATMENT INSIDE INFORMATIONAL AND SOCIAL PROTECTION SETTINGS

Adolescents and young people standing up to weight-related attack should have the alternative to search for course and comfort inside informative and therapeutic administrations settings. Because of the noteworthy activity of teachers and restorative administrations providers and their advancing contact with youth, both would large be able to influence overweight youth.

In any case, considers have suggested that a couple of educators and restorative administrations providers may have negative points of view concerning obesity that can interfere with their ability to give overweight youth the help that they may require.

My assessment bundle explored weight- related mindsets among 115 focus school and auxiliary educators and school prosperity workers.

Approximately one fifth of the school staff conveyed the view that obesity individuals are progressively excited, less perfect, less slanted to win pounding ceaselessly, and have surprising characters in contrast with no Hefty individuals. Around one fourth of the respondents considered fat to be as having more family issues than no enormous individuals and agreed with the declaration, "One of the most discernibly dreadful things that could happen to an individual would be for him/her to get obesity".

Strong contrary inclinations toward chunky individuals have been found among school understudies got together with physical guidance or exercise science programs. Given that a critical number of these school understudies will become physical preparing instructors, this finding has huge repercussions for youth: Antiquated irregularity inclinations among physical guidance staff could be a hindrance to joy or commitment in physical development among overweight and fat children and youngsters.

Despite affecting inter~ exercises with overweight understudies, school staffs guarantee attitudes about weight may in like manner sway the general school condition by coordinating whether the staff will intervene when weight criticize by various understudies occurs.

Similar contrary attitudes and speculations toward Chubby individuals have been found among various social affairs of prosperity specialists, including orderlies, dietitians and dietetic understudies, and specialists and clinical understudies similarly as investigators and other prosperity specialists invest critical energy in obesity treatment and shirking.

In an examination that investigated specialists' mindsets toward fat patients, most of the 620 specialists checked on considered huge to be as safe, appalling, and horrendous.

There is some verification that this relic favoritism may impact the thought that prosperity specialists give. For example, an examination that researched specialists' potential treatment of overweight patients using case reports of patients that differentiated remarkably in weight found that specialists declared that they would feel progressively negative toward overweight patients and that they would contribute less vitality with them.

Albeit little is pondered how the antique inclination of social protection master's persuasions teenagers' human administrations searching for direct, different assessments have found that fat women are more likely than no huge women to drop or delay therapeutic administrations courses of action, particularly for preventive organizations, for instance, chest and gynecological screening tests. Limits for searching for appropriate social protection recognized by corpulent women consolidate discourteous treatment, embarrassment at being checked or about their weight, negative mindsets of providers, unconstrained admonishment to get fit as a fiddle, and clinical equipment that is close to nothing.

On the other hand, an examination that investigated adult patients' reports of the level of care that they got from their primary care physicians found that lone overweight men uncovered that specialists contributed less vitality with them than with ordinary weight men; overweight women didn't report getting a lower level of care. Further assessment is relied upon to assess how negative mindsets inside the prosperity purposes for living impact the thought provided for grown-up similarly as youth peoples.

Given that therapeutic administrations providers and educators have open entryways for outfitting overweight youth with assistance and bearing concerning strong weight the official's practices, methods to improve the social protection and informational experiences of overweight adolescents and youngsters are meriting examination.

Some suggested changes for the people who treat or educate huge adolescents and young people fuse improved perception of the various sorts of disgrace that overweight youth endure, acknowledgment with organize resources open to youth, and moving toward youth with respect and compassion.

Proposed changes that are unequivocal to human administrations specialists fuse improved data on multidisciplinary prescriptions and making progressively open conditions for Fat youth by giving armless seats and greater evaluation outfits.

In view of our own assessment, in which we found that the majority of overweight youth have experienced weight deprecating, we would furthermore suggest that social protection providers approach an overweight adolescent under the doubt that the child has been the loss of a weight misuse and is tricky to comments about their weight.

Regardless of the way that it may be basic to discuss the clinical focal points of being at a sound weight, the conversation ought to consider the child's affectability to weight-related comments and fuse some helpful words about the child's appearance and other individual characteristics. It may be more brilliant to focus on procedures for social change instead of weight change, and the moves inborn to the two sorts of changes should be really discussed.

Finally, time should be taken to discuss weight-related maltreatment experiences and techniques for adjusting and responding to such events. Adolescents and young people need to understand that paying little psyche to their size; they should not be manhandled by anyone because of their weight.

MENTAL AFTEREFFECTS OF OBESITY AND WEIGHT-RELATED DERISION

Considering the unavoidable weight-related belittling looked by various overweight youth, differentiates in mental concerns might be imagined. At the present time delineate relationship among weight and overall mental worries, for instance, certainty and distress. In addition, we review a segment of the investigation that has examined connection between weight ridicule and mental outcomes.

CERTAINTY

Certainty is influenced by one's perceptions about how others regard and treat one. The past discussion obviously shows that various overweight youth see that others make negative assumptions about them and treat them contrastingly because of their weight. Thusly, we may plan to find immense complexities in certainty among overweight and non-overweight youth.

In addition, we may would like to find more grounded relationship among youngsters than among adolescents, given that appearance, fitting in with the norm, and social coordinated efforts will as a rule is key issues among this age gathering. In a review of the composing taking a gander at relationship among obesity and certainty among children and youngsters, French et al discovered more grounded relationship among adolescents then among kids. Regardless, revelations were not dependable across considers.

No examinations uncovered progressively huge degrees of trust in obesity youth than in no Fat youth. Results from the couple of arranged examinations that were investigated by French et al. we're clashing. Disclosures from later masses based examinations are furthermore somewhat clashing. An ongoing report that followed a colossal case of essential more youthful understudies developed 5 to 10 years at standard for quite a while found that weight was unfavorably associated with certainty at both measure and advancement.

This relationship was more grounded at advancement, suggesting that risk of low certainty is higher for overweight youngsters than for adolescents. Disclosures from a second fast approaching assessment including a huge case of youth moreover suggest that age may coordinate the relationship among overweight and certainty.

Certainty scores were not out and out interesting among 9-to 10-years-old Fat and no fat youths, while there were gigantic differentiations 4 years sometime later. This assessment furthermore found that ethnicity may coordinate this alliance: Certainty was conflictingly associated with weight status in Hispanic and Caucasian pre-grown-up youngsters anyway not in African American young women.

Still another assessment found that certainty is lower in overweight young people yet just if the effect of self-observation isn't controlled for. Thusly, disclosures from observational research suggest that weight will when all is said in done be connected with lower certainty, particularly in youngsters, anyway affiliations will all in all be unassuming and clashing across considers.

Additional exploration that examines connection between various spaces of certainty (e.g., athletic, social, appearance) and weight status may be relied upon to help uncover potential differences in certainty among overweight and no overweight youth.

OFFERING ASSISTANCE FOR OVERWEIGHT INDIVIDUALS

Family members of overweight youth similarly as educators, restorative administrations providers, and sidekicks can offer assistance in adjusting to weight-related destroying to lessen its idle limit influence on psychosocial thriving. Sponsorship from these key individuals is also expected to empower overweight youth to choose strong lifestyle choices that will prevent superfluous weight gain (e.g., getting normal physical activity, reducing television seeing).

Two masses based examinations found that overweight youngsters who had consistent families were more grounded and should psychosocial results than overweight adolescents whose families were less solid. Overweight adolescents brought up in solid families, in which family members swear off contribution negative comments about the child's appearance and weight, will breathe a sigh of relief pondering them and be increasingly disinclined to persevere through the psychosocial results related with being overweight. At the same time, gatherings of overweight children need to give openings and sensitive help to great dieting and physical development.

The concordance between these messages may present troubles for watchmen. A huge procedure that should be explored is the arrangement of privately settled intercessions that mean to help watchmen with walking this scarcely conspicuous distinction to propel their youths' prosperity. The investigation disclosures from our own gathering and various assessments have provoked the improvement of four establishments for gatekeepers who need to empower their adolescents to have a sound self-discernment and a strong body weight and structure the explanation behind a youngster raising book.

The four establishments are:

- Model sound practices for your adolescents,

- Provide a circumstance that makes it basic for your adolescents to choose steady choices,

- Focus less on weight and more on direct and all around prosperity, and,

- Provide a consistent circumstance with heaps of talking and extensively all the all the more tuning in.

More thought ought to be composed toward the gatekeepers of children and youngsters to help them with helping their children. Gatekeepers live in a comparative world as their children and are introduced to comparative weight-related weights. Watchmen may be stressed over the physical and mental flourishing of their youths, particularly in case they are overweight, and need instruments for supporting and not baffling their children's undertakings to grasp animating practices, such as themselves, and live profitable and fulfilling lives. As discussed already, some human administrations providers and instructors hold negative attitudes concerning obesity that can interfere with their ability to act in a consistent manner toward overweight patients and understudies.

Regardless, the majority of human administrations providers and teachers don't hold negative mindsets and are enthused about making sense of how they can be continuously solid.

At social events and get-togethers, clinicians as often as possible ask authorities how best to work with the overweight children and youngsters that they find in their practices, and meeting gatherings on this subject will when all is said in done be well known and especially participate. In an audit of school staff, our investigation bundle found that the majority of school-based human administrations providers and educators were enthused about setting off to a staff planning on the balance of weight-related agitating impacts.

Material on the most ideal approach to hinder weight destroying and how to propel the psychosocial flourishing of overweight youth could obviously be united into such gatherings Suggested practices join self-appraisal of their own weight-related viewpoints and experiences growing up, dispersing of exact real factors about the pernicious results of weight goading among youth, and unmistakable confirmation of ways to deal with inspect and advance sound weight-related practices in a fragile manner. A gadget that we have used in our trainings with school staff to help them with exploring their weight related favoritisms is the Irrefutable Association Test, which is an arranged word portrayal task planned to uncover comprehended weight inclinations.

New Moves, a school-based program for overweight youngsters or youngsters at risk for getting overweight on account of low degrees of physical activity, depends in transit of reasoning that overweight youth require a consistent and enduring condition to grasp sound weight-related practices. New Moves hopes to:

    Bring about positive change in physical development and eating practices to improve weight status and overall prosperity,

- Help youngsters work in a thin masterminded society and such as themselves, and,

- Help youngsters avoid heartbreaking weight control rehearses. Beginning revelations indicated that the program was by and large invited by youthful youngsters, their people, and the school staff.

In any case, beginning disclosures furthermore showed a necessity for an undeniably heightened, multicomponent intervention and a continuously broad appraisal to perceive an adjustment in social and physical outcomes. New Moves has been reevaluated and now consolidates a raised mediation stage in which youngsters look into an all-female physical instructional course with gatherings on sustenance, physical activity, and self-discernment and a help stage that fuses step by step social occasions over lunch.

The youngsters moreover look into solitary exhorting gatherings with Another Moves tutor all through the two times of the examination. During these gatherings, the New Moves guides set up a no irate and consistent environment in which the youngsters feel extraordinary talking about their experiences and challenges in endeavoring to change their weight-related practices. We are evaluating the New Moves program in a randomized controlled primer with 12 optional schools in Minnesota.

Obesity and weight tendency have been viewed as related with an assortment of troublesome psychosocial results in youth. Additional examination is relied upon to also clarify these affiliations. In their progressing total review of weight putting down in youth

Although additional examination is relied upon to also clarify these affiliations, mediations anticipated thwarting obesity and its psychosocial results are required now. Companions, school staff, restorative administrations specialists, and watchmen all fill in as critical concentrations for interventions anticipated decreasing weight destroying and growing help for youth overseeing weight related issues.

Additionally, intervention examines, surveying the impact of obesity contravention and treatment in youth, need to consolidate strong and expansive appraisal structures to assess program influence and to ensure that there are no unplanned pernicious effects on psychosocial results. It is basic to make and extensively realize intercessions that at the same time try to thwart both obesity and weight inclination among children and adolescents.

CHAPTER FIFTEEN: FREQUENTLY ASKED QUESTIONS

WOULD IT BE ADVISABLE FOR ME TO EXERCISE DURING STAGE 1?

Ordinary exercise is perhaps the best thing you can accomplish for your wellbeing, and doing some direct exercise will improve the weight-loss and medical advantages of Stage 1 of the diet. When in doubt, we urge you to proceed with your typical degree of activity and physical movement through the initial seven days of the Sirtfood Diet. Be that as it may, we recommend remaining inside your typical safe place, since delayed or excessively exceptional exercise may basically put a lot of weight on the body for this period. Tune in to your body. There's no compelling reason to push you to accomplish more exercise during Stage 1; let the Sirtfoods accomplish the difficult work.

I'M NOW THIN—WOULD I BE ABLE TO IN ANY CASE FOLLOW THE DIET?

We don't suggest Stage 1 of the Sirtfood Diet for any individual who is underweight. A decent method to see whether you are underweight is to compute your weight record or BMI. For whatever length of time that you know your tallness and weight, you can without much of a stretch decide this by utilizing one of the various BMI number crunchers on the web. In the event that your BMI is 18.5 or less, we don't suggest that you leave on Stage 1 of the diet.

In the event that your BMI is somewhere in the range of 18.5 and 20, we would at present urge alert, since following the diet may imply that your BMI falls underneath 18.5. While numerous individuals try to be super-thin, actually being underweight can contrarily influence numerous parts of wellbeing, adding to a brought down resistant framework, a raised danger of osteoporosis (debilitating of the bones), and fruitfulness issues. While we don't suggest Stage 1 of the diet on the off chance that you are underweight, we do in any case support the coordination of a lot of Sirtfoods into a decent method of eating so all the medical advantages of these nourishments can be procured.

Be that as it may, on the off chance that you are thin however have a BMI in the healthy range (20– 25), there is literally nothing preventing you from beginning. A lion's share of the members engaged with the pilot preliminary had BMIs in the healthy range, yet still lost great measures of weight and turned out to be increasingly conditioned. Critically, a considerable lot of them announced a huge improvement in vitality levels, essentialness, and appearance. Recall that the Sirtfood Diet is tied in with advancing wellbeing as much for what it's worth about getting in shape.

I'M CORPULENT—IS THE SIRTFOOD DIET DIRECTLY FOR ME?

Indeed! Try not to be put off by the way that lone a little minority of the members who set out on our pilot study were corpulent. This is on the grounds that the pilot study was done in a wellbeing and wellness club where individuals are commonly fitter and more wellbeing cognizant. Rather, be prodded on by the way that the rare sorts of people who were corpulent had stunningly better outcomes than our healthy-weight members. These outcomes have been reproduced by the great many individuals who have attempted the diet in reality. In view of the investigation into sirtuin actuation, you ought to likewise remain to harvest the best changes in your prosperity. Being corpulent builds the danger of various incessant medical issues, yet these are the very sicknesses that Sirtfoods help to ensure against.

I'VE ARRIVED AT MY OBJECTIVE WEIGHT AND WOULD PREFER NOT TO LOSE ANY MORE— DO I QUIT EATING SIRTFOODS?

In the first place, congrats on your weight-loss accomplishment! You've had incredible accomplishment with Sirtfoods, however it doesn't end now. While we don't suggest further calorie limitation, your diet should in any case give sufficient Sirtfoods. A significant number of our customers are currently at their optimal body structure however keeping on eating Sirtfood-rich diets. The incredible thing about Sirtfoods is that they are a lifestyle. The most ideal approach to consider them with respect to weight the board is that they help carry the body to the weight and synthesis it was intended to be. From here they work to keep up and keep you looking and feeling incredible. This is at last the objective we want for all Sirtfood Diet devotees.

I'VE COMPLETED STAGE 2—DO I QUIT DRINKING THE MORNING SIRTFOOD GREEN SQUEEZE NOW?

The green juice is our preferred method to get an awesome hit of Sirtfoods to begin the day, so we embrace it's drawn out utilization. Our Sirtfood green juice was deliberately intended to incorporate fixings that give a full range of sirtuin-actuating supplements in powerful fat-consuming and prosperity boosting dosages. In any case, we are totally supportive of assortment, and keeping in mind that we do suggest you proceed with a morning juice, we completely bolster anybody hoping to try different things with various Sirtfood juice creations.

I TAKE DRUG—IS IT ALRIGHT TO FOLLOW THE DIET?

The Sirtfood Diet is appropriate for a great many people, but since of its ground-breaking consequences for fat consuming and wellbeing, it can change certain malady forms and the activities of prescription recommended by your primary care physician. In like manner, certain drugs are not reasonable in a fasting state. During the preliminary of the Sirtfood Diet, we surveyed the appropriateness of every individual before the person in question left on the diet, particularly the individuals who were taking prescription. Clearly we can't do that for you, so on the off chance that you experience the ill effects of a huge medical issue, take endorsed meds, or have different motivations to be worried about setting out on the diet, we suggest you examine it with your primary care physician first. The odds are it will be ne and really of significant advantage for you, yet it's imperative to check.

WOULD I BE ABLE TO FOLLOW THE DIET IN CASE I'M PREGNANT?

We don't suggest leaving on the Sirtfood Diet on the off chance that you are attempting to consider or in the event that you are pregnant or breastfeeding. It is an incredible weight-loss diet, which makes it unacceptable. In any case, don't be put off eating a lot of Sirtfoods, since these are particularly healthy nourishments to incorporate as a component of a decent and differed diet for pregnancy. You will need to stay away from red wine, because of its liquor substance, and cutoff stimulated things, for example, espresso, green tea, and cocoa so as not to surpass 200 milligrams for each day of caffeine during pregnancy (one cup of moment espresso ordinarily contains around 100 milligrams of caffeine).

Proposals are not to surpass four cups of green tea every day and to stay away from match by and large. Other than that, you're allowed to receive the rewards of incorporating Sirtfoods in your diet. **ARE SIRTFOODS APPROPRIATE FOR YOUNGSTERS?**

The Sirtfood Diet is an amazing weight-loss diet and not intended for youngsters. In any case, that doesn't imply that youngsters should pass up the phenomenal medical advantages offered by incorporating more Sirtfoods in their general diet. A greater part of Sirtfoods speak to incredibly healthy nourishments for youngsters and assist them with accomplishing adjusted and nutritious diets. A large number of the plans intended for Stage 2 of the diet were made in light of families, including youngsters' taste buds. Any semblance of the Sirtfood pizza, the bean stew con carne, and the Sirtfood nibbles are flawless kid agreeable nourishments with a nutritional worth better than common food contributions for kids.

While most of Sirtfoods are very healthy for youngsters to eat, we don't suggest the green juice, which is excessively moved in fat consuming Sirtfoods. We additionally inform against noteworthy sources with respect to caffeine, for example, espresso and green tea. You will likewise should be cautious with the consideration of chilies and may pick to keep things milder for youngsters.

WILL I GET A MIGRAINE OR FEEL TIRED DURING STAGE 1?

Stage 1 of the Sirtfood Diet gives incredible normally happening food mixes in sums that the vast majority would not get in their ordinary diet, and certain individuals can respond as they adjust to this sensational nutritional change. This can incorporate manifestations, for example, a gentle migraine or tiredness, despite the fact that we would say these impacts are minor and brief.

Obviously, if side effects are serious or give you purpose behind concern, we suggest you look for brief clinical counsel. Having said that, we have seen nothing other than intermittent gentle manifestations that resolve rapidly, and inside a couple of days the vast majority finds they have a reestablished feeling of vitality, life, and prosperity.

WOULD IT BE A GOOD IDEA FOR ME TO TAKE ENHANCEMENTS?

Except if explicitly endorsed for you by your primary care physician or other social insurance proficient, we don't suggest aimless utilization of nutritional enhancements. You will ingest a huge and synergistic cluster of characteristic plant mixes from Sirtfoods, and it is these that will benefit you. You can't repeat these advantages with nutritional enhancements and, truth be told, some nutritional enhancements, for example, cell reinforcements, particularly whenever taken at high portions, may really meddle with the helpful impacts of Sirtfoods, which is the exact opposite thing you need.

At whatever point conceivable, we think it is vastly improved to get the supplements you need from eating a reasonable diet rich in Sirtfoods than from taking supplements in pill structure. Vegetarians will, in any case, have extraordinary nutritional contemplations, and our particular proposals for those following absolutely plant-based diets. Also, in light of the fact that plant proteins are lower in leucine, the amino corrosive that upgrades the activities of Sirtfoods, we have discovered that vegetarians can profit by enhancing their diet with an appropriate veggie lover protein powder. This especially applies to those taking part in elevated levels of activity. This enhancement ought to be taken at a different time of day from the Sirtfood green juice.

HOW REGULARLY WOULD I BE ABLE TO REHASH STAGES 1 AND 2?

Stage 1 can be rehashed on the off chance that you sense that you need a weight-loss or wellbeing help. To guarantee that there are no drawn out negative impacts to your digestion from calorie limitation, you should hold up in any event a month prior to rehashing. Be that as it may, we really locate that the vast majority need to rehash it no more regularly than once like clockwork probably and keep on getting astounding outcomes. Rather, in the event that you find you've gone off course, need some ne-tuning, or need more Sirtfood force, we suggest rehashing a few or the entire days of the Stage 2 area as regularly as you like. All things considered, Stage 2 is tied in with setting up a lifelong method of eating. Keep in mind, the magnificence of the Sirtfood Diet is that it doesn't expect you to feel like you are interminably on a tight eating routine, yet rather is the springboard to creating lifelong positive dietary changes that make a lighter, less fatty, more advantageous you.

DOES THE SIRTFOOD DIET Give ENOUGH FIBER?

Numerous Sirtfoods are normally rich in fiber. Onions, endive, and pecans are striking sources, with buckwheat and Medjool dates truly sticking out, implying that a Sirtfood-rich diet doesn't miss the mark in the fiber office. In any event, during Stage 1, when food utilization is diminished, the greater part of us will at present be devouring a fiber amount we are utilized to, particularly on the off chance that we pick the plans that contain buckwheat, beans, and lentils from the menu choices. In any case, for others known to be vulnerable to gut issues like clogging without higher fiber admissions, during Stage 1, particularly Days 1 to 3, an appropriate fiber supplement can be viewed as which ought to be examined with your medicinal services proficient.

I'VE FOUND OUT ABOUT SUPER NOURISHMENTS—WOULD IT BE ADVISABLE FOR ME TO INCORPORATE THESE IN MY DIET AS WELL?

The main thing you have to think about the term super food is that it's anything but a logical term at everything except a showcasing motto. You don't have to worry about supposed super nourishments on the grounds that the Sirtfood Diet unites the most advantageous food sources on earth into a progressive better approach for eating. Similarly as it is a slip-up to depend on taking a straightforward nutrient pill to make us healthy, so too it is a mix-up to depend on a solitary super food to do likewise. It is the entire diet, comprised of a wide range of Sirtfoods and their huge range of normal mixes, acting in cooperative energy that is the genuine mystery to accomplishing weight loss and lifelong wellbeing.

DO I NEED TO DO STAGE 1 FOR SEVEN DAYS— WOULD I BE ABLE TO DO LESS?

There's nothing otherworldly about Stage 1 being seven days. It is basically what we chose for our preliminary. We picked that since it was long enough to get amazing outcomes, however not all that long that it got difficult. It likewise fits perfectly into individuals' lives. Seven days is what was tried and what is demonstrated to be compelling. In any case, if for reasons unknown you find that you have to stop it by a day or two, do as such by finishing up to the finish of Day 5 or Day 6. Try not to stress; you will at present harvest a lot of the advantages.

WOULD I BE ABLE TO EAT ANYTHING I DESIRE ONCE I EAT A LOT OF SIRTFOODS AND STILL GET RESULTS?

One of the key reasons the Sirtfood Diet works so well long haul is that it advances great food as opposed to deriding awful food. Diets of rejection basically don't work long haul. The facts confirm that handled nourishments that are high in sugars and fats lessen sirtuin movement in the body, and in this manner a high utilization will diminish the advantages of Sirtfoods. In any case, on the off chance that you maintain your emphasis on expending a diet rich in Sirtfoods, in our experience you will find that you are charmingly fulfilled and will have less want for those prepared nourishments and wind up devouring far less garbage than the normal individual accordingly. On the off chance that you do at times wind up enjoying these handled nourishments, don't stresses over it—the intensity of Sirtfoods the remainder of the time will ensure you despite everything receive the rewards?

WOULD I BE ABLE TO EAT THE SAME NUMBER

OF SIRTFOODS, EVEN THE UNHEALTHY ONES, AS I LIKE AND STILL GET THINNER?

Truly! Keep in mind, calories and the drive to tally them is present day "headway." Over the way of life and incalculable ages that have profited by Sirtfoods, such an idea didn't exist, and there basically was no need. Individuals ate as they felt like it, and remained thin and liberated from infection. Given Sirtfoods' consequences for managing digestion and hunger, you just don't have to stress over eating an excessive number of them.

While this isn't a solicitation to an everything you-can-eat challenge, don't hesitate to eat as much Sirtfood as you like to fulfill your regular hunger. Our one special case is Medjool dates. Their consideration exhibits how high-sugar nourishments don't need to be terrible for you when eaten in the structure nature planned, and with some restraint. Be that as it may, control is critical to making dates a faultless liberal treat. Regarding drinks, with regards to red wine utilization, it's a given it ought to be flushed dependably and securely inside government proposals.

IS NATURAL BETTER?

In a perfect world, we would urge you to pick natural produce where conceivable, functional, and moderate. While there is little proof that degrees of ordinary nutrients and minerals contrast among natural and nonorganic produce, shouldn't something be said about the sirtuin-enacting supplements?

All things considered, natural produce conveys a more extravagant substance of sirtuin-initiating supplements. Recollect that the sirtuin-enacting polyphenols found in plant nourishments are delivered because of natural burdens, and without the extreme utilization of pesticides, naturally developed produce should fight that a lot harder to dissuade and avoid ecological predators.

This is probably going to bring about more significant levels of polyphenols being created, making natural produce conceivably a more remarkable Sirtfood than its nonorganic proportional. While natural is best, you will in any case get extraordinary outcomes from the Sirtfood Diet on the off chance that you select nonorganic produce. Natural is only the wonderful finish.

CHAPTER SIXTEEN: RECIPES

Some significant notes about these plans:

The plans indicate Thai chilies (otherwise called bird's-eye chilies). On the off chance that you have never attempted them, they are outstandingly more smoking than ordinary chilies. On the off chance that you are not used to hot food, we recommend beginning with a milder stew, for example, Serrano, adjusting the sum to suit your taste. As you get progressively familiar with normally incorporating chilies in your diet, you may find that you begin to appreciate more sweltering assortments, so please don't hesitate to try.

Miso is tasty flavor-stuffed aged soybean glue. You will discover it arrives in a scope of hues, ordinarily white, yellow, red, and earthy colored. The lighter-shaded miso glues are better than the dull ones, which can be very salty. For our plans, earthy colored or red miso will function admirably, however by all methods trial and see which flavor you like. Red miso will in general be the saltier of these, so in the event that you select this one, you may like to utilize somewhat less of it. The flavor and saltiness of miso can likewise shift between brands, so the best wager is check whatever type you purchase and alter the sum you use in like manner, so it's not very overwhelming. That implies a little experimentation, yet you'll before long get its hang.

- If you haven't cooked buckwheat previously, it couldn't be simpler. We suggest that you first completely wash the buckwheat in a strainer before putting it in a dish of bubbling water. Cooking times can fluctuate, so check the guidelines on your bundle.
- Flat-leaf parsley would be best for all the dishes, however in the event that you can't get hold of it, wavy will do.
- Onions, garlic, and ginger are constantly stripped except if

in any case expressed.

Salt and pepper are not utilized in these plans; however don't hesitate to season with ocean salt and dark pepper to your own taste inclinations. Sirtfoods offer such a large number of flavors, you will probably discover you don't require as much as you typically use. The expansion of dark pepper to any dish that contains turmeric is strongly suggested, as it will help increment the retention of its key sirtuin initiating supplement, curcumin.

ASIAN SHRIMP SAUTEED FOOD WITH BUCKWHEAT NOODLES

SERVES 1

1/3 pound (150g) shelled crude kind sized shrimp, deveined

2   teaspoons tamari (or soy sauce, on the off chance that you are not evading gluten) 2 teaspoons additional virgin olive oil
3   ounces (75g) soba (buckwheat noodles) 2 garlic cloves, cleaved
1 Thai bean stew, hacked

1 teaspoon cleaved new ginger 1/8 cup (20g) red onions cut
1/2 cup (45g) celery including leaves, cut and cut, with leaves put in a safe spot 1/2 cup (75g) green beans, cleaved 3/4 cup (50g) kale, generally hacked
1/2 cup (100ml) chicken stock

Cook the noodles in bubbling water for 5 to 8 minutes or as coordinated on the bundle. Channel and put in a safe spot.
Include the shrimp, noodles, and celery leaves to the dish, heat back to the point of boiling, at that point expel from the warmth and serve.

MISO AND SESAME COATED TOFU WITH GINGER AND STEW PAN-SEARED GREENS

SERVES 1

1 tablespoon miring

31/2 teaspoons (20g) miso glue

1 x 5-ounce (150g) square of firm tofu

1 stems (40g) celery, cut (around 1/3 cup when cut) 1/4 cup (40g) red onion, cut
1 little (120g) zucchini (around 1 cup when cut) Thai bean stew
Garlic cloves

Teaspoon nely cleaved new ginger 3/4 cup (50g) kale, cleaved
Teaspoons sesame seeds
1/4 cup (35g) buckwheat Teaspoon ground turmeric
Teaspoons additional virgin olive oil

1 teaspoon tamari (or soy sauce, on the off chance that you are not dodging gluten) Line a little broiling skillet with material paper.
Combine the miring and miso. Cut the tofu lengthways, and afterward cut each piece slantingly down the middle into triangles. Spread the tofu with the miso blend and leave to marinate while you set up different fixings.
Cut the celery, red onion, and zucchini on the edge. Finely slash the bean stew, garlic, and ginger and put in a safe spot.
Cook the kale in a liner for 5 minutes. Expel and put in a safe spot.

Spot the tofu in the simmering container, sprinkle the sesame seeds over the tofu, and dish in the broiler for 15 to 20 minutes, until pleasantly caramelized.
Wash the buckwheat in a sifter, at that point place in a container

of bubbling water alongside the turmeric. Cook as per the bundle guidelines, at that point channel.

Warmth the oil in a skillet; when hot include the celery, onion, zucchini, stew, garlic, and ginger and fry on high warmth for 1 to 2 minutes, at that point lessen to medium warmth for 3 to 4 minutes until the vegetables are cooked through yet at the same time crunchy. You may need to include a tablespoon of water if the vegetables begin to adhere to the skillet. Include the kale and tamari and cook for one more moment.

At the point when the tofu is prepared, present with the greens and buckwheat.

TURKEY ESCALOPE WITH SAGE, ESCAPADES, AND PARSLEY AND SPICED CAULIFLOWER "COUSCOUS"

Slight cutlets are ideal, yet in the event that you can just find turkey bosom, there are two different ways to transform it into an escalope. Contingent upon how thick the bosom is, you can either utilize a meat tenderizer, a sledge, or a moving pin to pound the steak until it is around 1/4 inch (5mm) thick. Or then again, on the off chance that you feel the bosom is unreasonably thick for this to work and you have a consistent hand, cut the bosom down the middle on a level plane and afterward pound each piece with the tenderizer.

SERVES 1

11/2 cups (150g) caulis bloom, generally hacked 2 garlic cloves, nely slashed

1/4 cup (40g) red onion, nely slashed 1 Thai bean stew, nely hacked

1 teaspoon nely slashed new ginger

2 tablespoons additional virgin olive oil 2 teaspoons ground turmeric

1/2 cup (30g) sun-dried tomatoes, nely cleaved 1/4 cup (10g)

new parsley, cleaved

1/3 pound (150g) turkey cutlet or steak (see above) 1 teaspoon dried sage juice of 1/4 lemon

1 tablespoon escapades

To make the "couscous," place the crude caulis bloom in a food processor. Heartbeat in 2-second but firsts to nely hack the caulis blossom until it looks like couscous. On the other hand, you can simply utilize a blade and cleave it nely.

Fry the garlic, red onion, bean stew, and ginger in 1 teaspoon of the oil until delicate however not caramelized. Include the turmeric and caulis bloom and cook for 1 moment. Expel from warmth and include the sun-dried tomatoes and a large portion of the parsley.

Coat the turkey escalope in the savvy and a little oil, and afterward utilize remaining oil to sear in a griddle over medium warmth for 5 to 6 minutes, turning normally.

At the point when cooked through, include the lemon juice, remaining parsley, tricks, and 1 tablespoon of water to the container. This will make a sauce to present with the caulis rose.

KALE AND RED ONION DAL WITH BUCKWHEAT
SERVES 1

1 teaspoon additional virgin olive oil Teaspoon mustard seeds

1/4 cup (40g) red onion, nely cleaved Garlic cloves, nely cleaved

1 teaspoon nely cleaved new ginger 1 Thai bean stew, nely slashed

1 Teaspoon gentle curry powder (medium or hot, on the off chance that you like) 2 Teaspoons ground turmeric

11/4 Cups (300ml) vegetable stock or water 1/4 Cup (40g) red lentils, washed

3/4 Cup (50g) kale, cleaved

31/2 Tablespoons (50ml) tinned coconut milk 1/3 Cup (50g) buckwheat

Warmth the oil in a medium pot over medium warmth and include the mustard seeds. As the mustard seeds begin to pop, include the onion, garlic, ginger, and bean stew. Cook for around 10 minutes, until delicate.

Include the curry powder and 1 teaspoon of the turmeric and cook the flavors for two or three minutes. Add the stock and heat to the point of boiling. Add the lentils to the skillet and stew for a further 25 to 30 minutes until the lentils are cooked through and you have a smooth dal.

Include the kale and coconut milk and cook for 5 minutes more.

In the meantime, cook the buckwheat as indicated by the bundle directions with the rest of the teaspoon of turmeric. Channel and serve close by the dal.

FRAGRANT CHICKEN BOSOM WITH KALE AND RED ONIONS AND A TOMATO AND STEW SALSA
SERVES 1

1/4 pound (120g) skinless, boneless chicken bosom 2 teaspoons ground turmeric juice of 1/4 lemon
1 tablespoon extra-virgin olive oil 3/4 cup (50g) kale, slashed
1/8 cup (20g) red onion, cut

1 teaspoon slashed new ginger 1/3 cup (50g) buckwheat
FOR THE SALSA

1 medium tomato (130g)

1 Thai bean stew, nely slashed

1 tablespoon escapades, nely slashed 2 tablespoons (5g) parsley, nely hacked juice of 1/4 lemon Blend in with the stew, tricks, parsley, and lemon juice. You could place everything in a blender; however the final product is somewhat extraordinary.
Marinate the chicken bosom in 1 teaspoon of the turmeric, the

lemon juice, and a little oil. Leave for 5 to 10 minutes.

Warmth an ovenproof griddle until hot, at that point include the marinated chicken and cook for a moment or so on each side, until pale brilliant, at that point move to the broiler (place on a preparing plate if your dish isn't ovenproof) for 8 to 10 minutes or until cooked through. Expel from the broiler, spread with foil, and leave to rest for 5 minutes before serving.

In the interim, cook the kale in a liner for 5 minutes. Fry the red onions and the ginger in a little oil, until delicate yet not seared, at that point include the cooked kale and fry for one more moment. Cook the buckwheat as indicated by the bundle directions with the rest of the teaspoon of turmeric. Serve nearby the chicken, vegetables, and salsa.

HARISSA HEATED TOFU WITH CAULIFLOWER "COUSCOUS"

SERVES 1

3/8 cup (60g) red ringer pepper

1 Thai bean stew, split 2 garlic cloves around 1 tablespoon extra-virgin olive oil spot of ground cumin touch of ground coriander juice of 1/4 lemon
7 ounces (200g) tofu

13/4 cups (200g) caulis bloom, generally slashed 1/4 cup (40g) red onion, nely slashed
1 teaspoon nely slashed new ginger Teaspoons ground turmeric
1/2 cup (30g) sun-dried tomatoes, nely cleaved 1/2 cup (20g) parsley, cleaved

To make the harissa, cut the red pepper the long way around the center so you have decent at cuts, evacuate any seeds, at that point place in a cooking skillet with the bean stew and one of the garlic cloves. Hurl with a little oil and the dried cumin and coriander and dish in the stove for 15 to 20 minutes until the peppers are delicate however not very cooked. (Leave the broiler on at this setting.) Cool, and afterward mix in a food processor with the lemon juice until smooth.

Cut the tofu lengthways and afterward cut every half slantingly into triangles. Spot in a little nonstick broiling container or one fixed with material paper, spread with the harissa, and meal in the stove for 20 minutes—the tofu ought to have consumed the marinade and turned dim red.

To make the "couscous," place the crude cauliflower in a food processor. Heartbeat in 2-second bursts to nely hack the caulis bloom until it looks like couscous. On the other hand, you can simply utilize a blade and hack it nely.

Mince the rest of the garlic clove. Fry the garlic, red onion, and ginger in 1 teaspoon of the oil, until delicate however not sautéed, at that point include the turmeric and caulis bloom and cook for 1 moment.

Expel from warmth and mix in the sun-dried tomatoes and parsley. Present with the heated tofu.

SIRT MUESLI

In the event that you need to make this in mass or set it up the prior night, just consolidate the dry fixings and store the blend in an impermeable compartment. All you have to do the following day is include the strawberries and yogurt and it's all set.
SERVES 1

1/4 cup (20g) buckwheat pieces

3 tablespoons (15g) coconut pieces or dried coconut 1/4 cup (40g) Medjool dates, hollowed and cleaved 1/8 cup (15g) pecans, cleaved
11/2 tablespoons (10g) cocoa nibs

2/3 cup (100g) strawberries, hulled and cleaved

3/8 cup (100g) plain Greek yogurt (or veggie lover elective, for example, soy or coconut yogurt) Combine the entirety of the fixings (forget about the strawberries and yogurt if not serving immediately).

SEARED SALMON FILET WITH CARAMELIZED ENDIVE, ARUGULA, AND CELERY LEAF SERVING OF MIXED GREENS

SERVES 1

1/4 cup (10g) parsley juice of 1/4 lemon 1 tablespoon tricks

1 clove garlic, generally hacked Tablespoon extra-virgin olive oil

1/4 avocado, stripped, stoned, and diced 2/3 cup (100g) cherry tomatoes split

1/8 cup (20g) red onion daintily cut 13/4 ounces (50g) arugula Tablespoons (5g) celery leaves

X 5-ounce (150g) skinless salmon fillet Teaspoons earthy colored sugar

1 head of endive, around 21/2 ounces (70g), split lengthways

For the dressing, place the parsley, lemon juice, tricks, garlic, and 2 teaspoons of the oil in a food processor or blender and mix until smooth.

For the plate of mixed greens, blend the avocado, tomato, and red onion, arugula, and celery leaves together.

Warmth a skillet over high Temperature. Focus on the salmon a little oil and singe it in the hot prospect minute or so to caramelize the outside of the sh. Move to a preparing plate and spot in the stove for 5 to 6 minutes or until cooked through; diminish the cooking time by 2 minutes on the off chance that you like your fish served pink inside.

In the interim, clear out the skillet and spot it back on high warmth. Blend the earthy colored sugar in with the rest of the teaspoon of oil and brush it over the cut sides of the endive. Spot the endive chop sides down in the hot container and cook for 2 to 3 minutes, turning consistently, until delicate and pleasantly caramelized everywhere. Prepare the plate of mixed greens in the dressing and present with the salmon and endive.

SAUTÉED SALMON FILET WITH CARAMELIZED ENDIVE, ARUGULA, AND CELERY LEAF PLATE OF MIXED GREENS

SERVES 1

1/4 cup (10g) parsley juice of 1/4 lemon 1 tablespoon escapades
1 clove garlic, generally slashed Tablespoon extra-virgin olive oil
1/4 avocado, stripped, stoned, and diced 2/3 cup (100g) cherry tomatoes, divided 1/8 cup (20g) red onion meagerly cut 13/4 ounces (50g) arugula
Tablespoons (5g) celery leaves

X 5-ounce (150g) skinless salmon filet Teaspoons earthy colored sugar
1 head of endive, around 21/2 ounces (70g), divided lengthways

For the dressing, place the parsley, lemon juice, escapades, garlic, and 2 teaspoons of the oil in a food processor or blender and mix until smooth.

For the serving of mixed greens, blend the avocado, tomato, and red onion, arugula, and celery leaves together.

Focus on the salmon a little oil and burn it in the hot search for gold moment or so to caramelize the outside of the sh. Move to a preparing plate and spot in the stove for 5 to 6 minutes or until cooked through; decrease the cooking time by 2 minutes on the off chance that you like your fish served pink inside.

In the interim, clear out the griddle and spot it back on high warmth. Blend the earthy colored sugar in with the rest of the teaspoon of oil and brush it over the cut sides of the endive. Spot the endive chop sides down in the hot dish and cook for 2 to 3 minutes, turning routinely, until delicate and pleasantly caramelized everywhere. Prepare the plate of mixed greens in the dressing and present with the salmon and endive.

TUSCAN BEAN STEW

SERVES 1

Tablespoon Additional Virgin Olive Oil 1/3 cup (50g) red onion, nely cleaved
1/4 cup (30g) carrot, stripped and nely hacked 1/3 cup (30g) celery, cut and nely hacked Garlic Cloves, Nely Hacked
1/2 Thai stew, nely cleaved (discretionary) 1 teaspoon herbs de Provence
7/8 cup (200ml) vegetable stock

1 x 14-ounce can (400g) hacked Italian tomatoes 1 teaspoon tomato purée
3/4 cup (130 g) canned blend beans (depleted weight) 3/4 cup (50g) kale, generally hacked
1 tablespoon generally hacked parsley 1/4 cup (40g) buckwheat
Spot the oil in a medium pot over low to medium warmth and delicately fry the onion, carrot, celery, garlic, bean stew (if utilizing), and herbs, until the onion is delicate however not sautéed.
Include the stock, tomatoes, and tomato purée and heat to the point of boiling. Include the beans and stew for 30 minutes.
Include the kale and cook for another 5 to 10 minutes, until delicate, at that point include the parsley.
In the interim, cook the buckwheat as per the bundle directions, channel, and afterward present with the stew.

MISO-MARINATED PREPARED COD WITH SAUTEED GREENS AND SESAME

SERVES 1

31/2 teaspoons (20g) miso 1 tablespoon miring
1 tablespoon extra-virgin olive oil X 7-ounce (200g) skinless cod

filet 1/8 cup (20g) red onion, cut

3/8 cup (40g) celery, cut Garlic cloves, finely hacked 1 Thai stew, finely hacked

1 teaspoon finely hacked new ginger 3/8 cup (60g) green beans

3/4 cup (50g) kale, generally hacked Teaspoon sesame seeds

Tablespoons (5g) parsley, generally hacked

1 tablespoon tamari (or soy sauce, in the event that you are not keeping away from gluten) 1/4 cup (40g) buckwheat

1 teaspoon ground turmeric

Blend the miso, miring, and 1 teaspoon of the oil. Rub everywhere throughout the cod and leave to marinate for 30 minutes.

Prepare the cod for 10 minutes.

In the interim, heat a huge griddle or wok with the rest of the oil. Include the onion and pan fried food for a couple of moments, at that point include the celery, garlic, stew, ginger, green beans, and kale. Hurl and fry until the kale is delicate and cooked through. You may need to add a little water to the dish to help the cooking procedure.

Cook the buckwheat as indicated by the bundle directions along with the turmeric.

Include the sesame seeds, parsley, and tamari to the sautéed food and present with the buckwheat and fish.

SOBA (BUCKWHEAT NOODLES) IN A MISO STOCK WITH TOFU, CELERY, AND KALE

SERVES 1

3 ounces (75g) soba (buckwheat noodles) Tablespoon extra-virgin olive oil

1/8 cup (20g) red onion, cut Garlic cloves, finely slashed

1 teaspoon finely slashed new ginger

11/4 cups (300ml) vegetable stock, in addition to some extra, if vital 13/4 tablespoons (30g) miso glue
3/4 cup (50g) kale, generally slashed 1/2 cup (50g) celery, generally slashed 1 teaspoon sesame seeds
31/2 ounces (100g) rm tofu, cut into 1/4-to 1/2-inch (0.5 to 1cm) shapes (around 3/8 cup)

1 teaspoon tamari (discretionary; or soy sauce, on the off chance that you are not maintaining a strategic distance from gluten)
Spot the noodles in a skillet of bubbling water and cook for 5 to 8 minutes or as indicated by the bundle directions.
Warmth the oil in a pot; include the onions, garlic, and ginger and fry over medium warmth in the oil, until delicate yet not sautéed. Include the stock and miso and heat to the point of boiling.
Add the kale and celery to the miso stock and stew tenderly for 5 minutes (do whatever it takes not to heat up the miso, as you will crush the flavor and cause it to go grainy in surface). You may need to include somewhat more stock as required.
Include the cooked noodles and sesame seeds and permit to warm through, at that point include the tofu. Serve in a bowl sprinkled with a little tamari, whenever wanted.

SIRT SUPER SERVING OF MIXED GREENS

SERVES 1
13/4 ounces (50g) arugula

13/4 ounces (50g) endive leaves

31/2 ounces (100g) smoked salmon cuts

1/2 cup (80g) avocado, stripped, stoned, and cut 1/2 cup (50g) celery including leaves, cut

1/8 cup (20g) red onion, cut 1/8 cups (15g) pecans, slashed 1 tablespoon escapades

1 enormous Medjool date, hollowed and cleaved 1 tablespoon extra-virgin olive oil juice of 1/4 lemon

1/4 cup (10g) parsley, slashed

Spot the serving of mixed greens leaves on a plate or in an enormous bowl. Combine all the rest of the fixings and serve on the leaves.

Varieties

For a lentil Sirt super plate of mixed greens, supplant the smoked salmon with 11/3 cups (100g) canned green lentils or cooked Le Puy lentils.

For a chicken Sirt super plate of mixed greens, supplant the smoked salmon with a cut cooked chicken bosom.

For a fish Sirt super plate of mixed greens, essentially supplant the smoked salmon with canned fish (in water or oil, as per inclination).

SINGE FLAME BROILED MEAT WITH A RED WINE JUS, ONION RINGS, GARLIC KALE, AND HERB-COOKED POTATOES

SERVES 1

1/2 cup (100g) potatoes, stripped and cut into 3/4-inch (2cm) diced pieces Tablespoon extra-virgin olive oil

Tablespoons (5g) parsley, finely cleaved

1/3 cup (50g) red onion, cut into rings 2 ounces (50g) kale, cut

2 garlic cloves, finely cleaved

1 x 4-to 5-ounce (120 to 150g) hamburger tenderloin (around 11/2 inches or 3.5cm thick) or sirloin steak (3/4 inch or 2cm thick)

3 tablespoons (40ml) red wine 5/8 cup (150ml) hamburger stock

1 teaspoon tomato purée

1 teaspoon corn our, broke down in 1 tablespoon water

Spot the potatoes in a pan of bubbling water, heat back to the point of boiling, and cook for 4 to 5 minutes, at that point channel. Spot in a cooking skillet with 1 teaspoon of the oil and meal in the hot stove for 35 to 45 minutes. Turn the potatoes each
10 minutes to guarantee in any event, cooking. At the point when cooked, expel from the broiler, sprinkle with the cleaved parsley, and blend well.

Fry the onion in 1 teaspoon of the oil over medium warmth for 5 to 7 minutes, until delicate and pleasantly caramelized. Keep warm.

Steam the kale for 2 to 3 minutes, at that point channel. Fry the garlic delicately in 1/2 teaspoon of oil for 1 moment, until delicate however not cooked. Include the kale and fry for 1 to 2 minutes more, until delicate. Keep warm.

Warmth an ovenproof griddle over high warmth until smoking. Coat the meat in 1/2 teaspoon of the oil and fry in the hot container over medium-high warmth as indicated by how you like your meat done (see our manual for the cooking times). On the off chance that you like your meat medium, it is smarter to burn it and afterward move the container to a broiler set at 425°F (220°C) and finish the cooking that path for the endorsed occasions.

Expel the meat from the skillet and put aside to rest. Add the wine to the hot skillet to raise any meat buildup. Stew to decrease the wine significantly, until sweet and with a concentrated flavor.

Include the stock and tomato purée to the steak dish and heat to the point of boiling, at that point add the corn-our glue to thicken your sauce, including it a little at once until you have your ideal consistency. Mix in any of the juices from the refreshed steak, and present with the broiled potatoes, kale, onion rings, and red wine sauce.

STEAK COOKING TIMES

11/2-INCH-THICK (3.5CM) TENDERLOIN

Blue: around 11/minutes each side Uncommon: around 21/minutes each side
Medium-uncommon: around 31/minutes each side Medium: around 41/minutes each side
/4-INCH-THICK (2CM) SIRLOIN STEAK

Blue: around 1 moment each side Uncommon: around 11/minutes each side
Medium-uncommon: around 2 minutes each side Medium: around 21/minutes each side

KIDNEY BEAN MOLE WITH HEATED POTATO

SERVES 1

1/4 cup (40g) red onion, nely cleaved Teaspoon nely cleaved new ginger Garlic cloves, nely cleaved
1 Thai bean stew, nely cleaved

1 teaspoon additional virgin olive oil

1 teaspoon ground turmeric 1 teaspoon ground cumin spot of ground clove touch of ground cinnamon
1 medium heating potato

7/8 cup (190g) canned cleave tomatoes

1 teaspoon earthy colored sugar

1/3 cup (50g) red ringer pepper, cored, seeds expelled, and generally hacked 5/8 cup (150ml) vegetable stock
1   tablespoon cocoa powder Teaspoon sesame seeds
Teaspoons nutty spread (smooth's if accessible, yet stout is ne)

168

7/8 cup (150g) canned kidney beans

2 tablespoons (5g) parsley, cleaved Warmth the broiler to 400°F (200°)

Fry the onion, ginger, garlic, and bean stew in the oil in a medium pan over medium warmth for around 10 minutes, or until delicate. Include the flavors and cook for a further 1 to 2 minutes. Spot the potato on a preparing plate in the hot broiler and heat for 45 to an hour, until delicate in center (or more, contingent upon how firm you like the outside).

In the interim, include the tomatoes, sugar, red pepper, stock, cocoa powder, sesame seeds, nutty spread, and kidney beans to the pan and stew delicately for 45 to an hour.

Sprinkle with the parsley to wrap up. Cut the potato down the middle and serve the mole on top.

SIRTFOOD OMELET

SERVES 1

Around 2 ounces (50g) cut smudgy bacon (or 2 rashers, smoked or standard, contingent upon your taste)

3 medium eggs

11/4 ounces (35g) red endive, daintily cut 2 tablespoons (5g) parsley, nely cleaved 1 teaspoon turmeric

1 teaspoon additional virgin olive oil

Warmth a nonstick skillet. Cut the bacon into flimsy strips and cook over high warmth until fresh. You don't have to include any oil, there is sufficient fat in the bacon to cook it. Expel from the container and spot on a paper towel to deplete any abundance fat. Wipe the skillet clean.

Whisk the eggs and blend in with the endive, parsley, and turmeric. Slash the cooked bacon into solid shapes and mix through the eggs.

Warmth the oil in the griddle—the skillet ought to be hot yet not smoking. Include the egg blend and, utilizing a spatula, move it around the container to begin to cook the egg. Keep the bits of cooked egg moving and whirl the crude egg around the skillet until the omelet level is even. Diminish the warmth and let the omelet firm up. Facilitate the spatula around the edges and overlay the omelet down the middle or move up and serve.

PREPARED CHICKEN BOSOM WITH PECAN AND PARSLEY PESTO AND RED ONION SERVING OF MIXED GREENS

SERVES 1

3/8 cup (15g) parsley 1/8 cup (15g) pecans
4 teaspoons (15g) Parmesan cheddar, ground

1 tablespoon extra-virgin olive oil juice of 1/2 lemon 3 tablespoons (50ml) water
51/2 ounces (150g) skinless chicken bosom 1/8 cup (20g) red onions, nely cut
1 teaspoon red wine vinegar 11/4 ounces (35g) arugula
2/3 cup (100g) cherry tomatoes split 1 teaspoon balsamic vinegar

To make the pesto, place the parsley, pecans, Parmesan, olive oil, a large portion of the lemon juice, and a tad bit of the water in a food processor or blender and mix until you have a smooth glue.

Include more water continuously until you have your favored consistency.

Marinate the chicken bosom in 1 tablespoon of the pesto and the rest of the lemon squeeze in the cooler for 30 minutes, longer if conceivable.

Preheat the broiler to 400°F (200°C).

Warmth an ovenproof griddle over medium-high warmth Fry the chicken in its marinade for 1 moment on either side, at that point move the dish to the stove and cook for 8 minutes, or until cooked through.

Marinate the onions in the red wine vinegar for 5 to 10 minutes. Channel the fluid.

At the point when the chicken is cooked, expel it from the stove, spoon another tablespoon of pesto over it, and let the warmth from the chicken liquefy the pesto.

Spread with foil and leave to rest for 5 minutes before serving.

Join the arugula, tomatoes, and onion and sprinkle with the balsamic vinegar. Present with the chicken, spooning over the rest of the pesto.

POTATO PLATE OF MIXED GREENS

SERVES 1

1 cup (100g) celery including leaves, generally cleaved 1/2 cup (50g) apple, generally cleaved

3/8 cup (50g) pecans, generally cleaved Tablespoon (10g) red onion, generally cleaved Tablespoons (5g) parsley, cleaved

1 tablespoon tricks

1 tablespoon extra-virgin olive oil 1 teaspoon balsamic vinegar juice of 1/4 lemon 1/4 teaspoon Dijon mustard around 2 ounces (50g) arugula around 11/2 ounces (35g) endive leaves

Blend the celery and its leaves, apple, pecans, and onion with the parsley and tricks.

In a bowl, whisk the oil, vinegar, lemon juice, and mustard to make the dressing. Serve the celery blend on the arugula and endive and shower with the dressing.

SIMMERED EGGPLANT WEDGES WITH PECAN AND PARSLEY PESTO AND TOMATO SERVING OF MIXED GREENS

SERVES 1

1/2 cup (20g) parsley 3/4 ounces (20g) pecans

1/8 cup (20g) Parmesan cheddar (or utilize a veggie lover or vegetarian elective), ground 1 tablespoon extra-virgin olive oil juice of 1/4 lemon

3 tablespoons (50ml) water

1 little eggplant (around 51/2 ounces or 150g), quartered 1/8 cup (20g) red onions cut

1 teaspoon (5ml) red wine vinegar 11/4 ounces (35g) arugula

2/3 cup (100g) cherry tomatoes 1 teaspoon (5ml) balsamic vinegar Warmth the stove to 400°F (200°C)

To make the pesto, place the parsley, pecans, Parmesan, olive oil, and a large portion of the lemon squeeze in a food processor or blender and mix until you have smooth glue. Include the water continuously until you have the right consistency — it ought to be sufficiently thick to adhere to the eggplant.

Brush the eggplant with a tad bit of the pesto, holding the rest to serve. Spot on a preparing plate and dish or 25 to 30 minutes, until the eggplant is brilliant earthy colored, delicate, and sodden. In the interim, spread the red onion with the red wine vinegar and put in a safe spot—this will mollify and improve the onion. Channel the vinegar before serving.

Consolidate the arugula, tomatoes, and depleted onion and shower the balsamic vinegar over the plate of mixed greens. Present with the hot eggplant, spooning the rest of the pesto over it.

SIRTFOOD SMOOTHIE

SERVES 1

3/8 cup (100g) plain Greek yogurt (or veggie lover elective, for example, soy or coconut yogurt) 6 pecan parts

8 to 10 medium strawberries, hulled bunch of kale, stalks expelled 3/4 ounce (20g) dull chocolate (85 percent cocoa solids) 1 Medjool date, pitted 1/2 teaspoon ground turmeric slender bit

(1 to 2mm) of Thai stew 7/8 cup (200ml) unsweetened almond milk

Rush all the fixings in a blender until smooth.

STUFFED ENTIRE WHEAT PITA

SERVES 1

Entire wheat pitas are an incredible method to pack a lot of Sirtfoods into a speedy lunch or helpful and convenient stuffed feast. You can mess with amounts and get inventive, at the end of the day everything you do is loading the fixings in and it's all set.

FOR A MEAT CHOICE

3 ounces (80g) cooked turkey cuts, slashed 3/4 ounce (20g) cheddar, diced

1/4 cup (35g) cucumber, diced 1/4 cup (35g) red onion, slashed 1 ounce (25g) arugula, slashed

11/2 to 2 tablespoons (10 to 15g) pecans, generally slashed FOR THE DRESSING

Tablespoons Extra-Virgin Olive oil1 tablespoon balsamic vinegar run of lemon juice

FOR A VEGGIE LOVER ALTERNATIVE

To 3 Tablespoons Hummus 1/4 cup (35g) cucumber, diced

1/4 cup (35g) red onion, cleaved 1 ounce (25g) arugula, cleaved

11/2 to 2 tablespoons (10 to 15g) pecans, generally cleaved

FOR THE VEGGIE LOVER DRESSING

1 tablespoon extra-virgin olive oil runs of lemon juice

BUTTERNUT SQUASH AND DATE TAGINE WITH

BUCKWHEAT SERVES 4

3 teaspoons additional virgin olive oil 1 red onion, nely slashed

1 tablespoon nely slashed new ginger 4 garlic cloves, nely slashed

2 Thai chilies, nely slashed 1 tablespoon ground cumin Cinnamon stick

Tablespoons ground turmeric

2 x 14-ounce jars (400g every one) of slashed tomatoes 11/4 cups (300ml) vegetable stock

2/3 cup (100g) Medjool dates, hollowed and cleaved

X 14-ounce can (400g) of chickpeas, depleted and washed

21/2 cups (500g) butternut squash, stripped and cut into scaled down pieces 11/4 cups (200g) buckwheat

Tablespoons (5g) new coriander, cleaved 1/4 cup (10g) new parsley, cleaved Warmth the stove to 400°F (200°C)

Fry the onion, ginger, garlic, and bean stew in two teaspoons of the oil for 2 to 3 minutes. Include the cumin and cinnamon and 1 tablespoon of the turmeric, and cook for another 1 to 2 minutes.

Include the tomatoes, stock, dates, and chickpeas and stew tenderly for 45 to an hour. You may need to include a little water every once in a while to accomplish a thick, clingy consistency and to ensure the container doesn't run dry.

Spot the squash in a cooking dish, hurl with the rest of the oil, and meal for 30 minutes until delicate and scorched around the edges.

Close to the finish of the tagine's cooking time, cook the buckwheat as indicated by the bundle guidelines with the rest of the tablespoon of turmeric*

Add the broiled squash to the tagine alongside the coriander and parsley and present with the buckwheat.

YOGURT WITH BLENDED BERRIES, SLASHED PECANS, AND DULL CHOCOLATE

SERVES 1

Around 11/3 cups (125g) blended berries

2/3 cup (150g) plain Greek yogurt (or veggie lover elective, for example, soy or coconut yogurt) 1/4 cup (25g) pecans, slashed 11/2 tablespoons (10g) dim chocolate (85 percent cocoa solids), ground Just add your favored berries to a bowl and top with the yogurt.
Sprinkle with the pecans and chocolate.

CHICKEN AND KALE CURRY WITH BOMBAY POTATOES

SERVES 4

4 x 41/2-to 51/2-ounce (120 to 150g) skinless, boneless chicken bosoms, cut into scaled down pieces 4 tablespoons additional virgin olive oil
3 tablespoons ground turmeric 2 red onions cut
Thai chilies, nely hacked Garlic cloves, nely hacked
1 tablespoon nely hacked new ginger
1 tablespoon gentle curry powder

X 14-ounce (400g) can chopped tomatoes 21/8 cups (500ml) chicken stock
7/8 cup (200ml) coconut milk Cardamom units
Cinnamon stick

11/3 pounds (600g) reddish brown potatoes 1/4 cup (10g) parsley, hacked
22/3 cups (175g) kale, hacked Tablespoons (5g) coriander, hacked
Focus on the chicken pieces 1 teaspoon of the oil and 1

tablespoon of the turmeric. Leave to marinate for 30 minutes.

Fry the chicken over high warmth (there ought to be sufficient oil in the marinade to cook the chicken) for 4 to 5 minutes until pleasantly sautéed all finished and cooked through, at that point expel from the dish and put in a safe spot.

Warmth 1 tablespoon of the oil in the griddle over medium warmth and include the onion, bean stew, garlic, and ginger. Fry for around 10 minutes, or until delicate, at that point include the curry powder and another tablespoon of the turmeric and cook for another 1 to 2 minutes. Add the tomatoes to the dish, and afterward let them cook for an additional 2 minutes. Include the stock, coconut milk, cardamom, and cinnamon stick and leave to stew for 45 to an hour. Check the container at customary interims to guarantee it doesn't run dry—you may need to include increasingly stock.

Warmth the stove to 425°F (220°C). While your curry is stewing, strip the potatoes and cut them into little pieces. Spot in bubbling water with the rest of the tablespoon of turmeric and bubble for 5 minutes. Channel well and permit steaming dry for 10 minutes. They ought to be white and flaky around the edges. Move to a cooking container, hurl with the rest of the oil, and meal for 30 minutes or until brilliant earthy colored and fresh. Hurl through the parsley when they're prepared.

At the point when the curry has your necessary consistency, include the kale, cooked chicken, and coriander and cook for an additional 5 minutes, to guarantee the chicken is cooked through, at that point present with the potatoes.

SPICED FRIED EGGS

SERVES 1

1 teaspoon additional virgin olive oil 1/8 cup (20g) red onion, nely slashed 1/2 Thai bean stew, nely hacked
3 medium eggs

1/4 cup (50ml) milk Teaspoon ground turmeric
Tablespoons (5g) parsley, nely hacked

Warmth the oil in a skillet and fry the red onion and stew until delicate however not caramelized. Whisk together the eggs, milk, turmeric, and parsley. Add to the hot dish and keep cooking over low to medium warmth, continually moving the egg blend around the skillet to scramble it and prevent it from staying/consuming.

At the point when you have accomplished your ideal consistency, serve.

SIRT BEAN STEW CON CARNE

SERVES 4

1 red onion, nely slashed

3 garlic cloves, nely slashed 2 Thai chilies, nely slashed
1 tablespoon extra-virgin olive oil 1 tablespoon ground cumin
1 tablespoon ground turmeric

1 pound (450g) lean ground hamburger (5 percent fat) 5/8 cup (150ml) red wine
Red chime pepper, cored, seeds evacuated and cut into scaled down pieces X 14-ounce (400g) jars hack tomatoes
1 tablespoon tomato purée Tablespoon cocoa powder
7/8 cup (150g) canned kidney beans 11/4 cups (300ml) meat stock Tablespoons (5g) new coriander, hacked 2 tablespoons (5g) new parsley, hacked 1 cup (160g) buckwheat
In a huge pot, fry the onion, garlic, and bean stew in the oil over medium warmth for 2 to 3 minutes, at that point include the flavors and cook for one more moment or two. Include the ground hamburger and cook for 2 to 3 minutes over medium-high warmth until the meat is pleasantly sautéed everywhere.

Include the red wine and permit it to rise to lessen it significantly.

Include the red pepper, tomatoes, tomato purée, cocoa, kidney beans, and stock and leave to stew for 60 minutes. You may need to include a little water occasionally to accomplish a thick, clingy consistency. Not long before serving, mix in the slashed herbs.

In the meantime, cook the buckwheat as indicated by the bundle directions and serve nearby the bean stew.

MUSHROOM AND TOFU SCRAMBLE

SERVES 1

31/2 ounces (100g) extra-firm tofu 1 teaspoon ground turmeric

1 teaspoon mellow curry powder

1/3 cup (20g) kale, generally slashed Teaspoon additional virgin olive oil 1/8 cup (20g) red onion meagerly cut 1/2 Thai bean stew, daintily cut

3/4 cup (50g) mushrooms, meagerly cut Tablespoons (5g) parsley, nely cleaved

Envelop the tofu by paper towels and spot something overwhelming on top to enable it to deplete. Blend the turmeric and curry powder and include a little water until you have accomplished light glue. Steam the kale for 2 to 3 minutes.

Warmth the oil in a griddle over medium warmth and fry the onion, bean stew, and mushrooms for 2 to 3 minutes until they have begun to brown and mellow.

Disintegrate the tofu into reduced down pieces and add to the skillet, pour the flavor blend over the tofu, and blend altogether. Cook over medium warmth for 2 to 3 minutes so the flavors are cooked through and the tofu has begun to brown.

Add the kale and keep on cooking over medium warmth for one more moment. At last, include the parsley, blend well, and serve.

SMOKED SALMON PASTA WITH STEW AND ARUGULA

SERVES 4

2 tablespoons additional virgin olive oil Red onion, nely hacked
Garlic cloves, nely hacked 2 Thai chilies, nely hacked
1 cup (150g) cherry tomatoes split 1/2 cup (100ml) white wine
9 to 11 ounces (250 to 300g) buckwheat pasta 9 ounces (250g) smoked salmon
2 tablespoons tricks juice of 1/2 lemon 2 ounces (60g) arugula
1/4 cup (10g) parsley, slashed
Warmth 1 teaspoon of the oil in a griddle over medium warmth. Include the onion, garlic, and bean stew and fry until delicate yet not caramelized.
Add the tomatoes and leave to cook for a moment or two. Include the white wine and air pocket to decrease considerably.
In the interim, cook the pasta in bubbling water with 1 teaspoon of the oil for 8 to 10 minutes relying upon how still somewhat firm you like it, and afterward channel.
Cut the salmon into strips and add to the container of tomatoes alongside the tricks, lemon juice, arugula, and parsley. Include the pasta, blend well, and serve right away. Sprinkle any outstanding oil over the top.

BUCKWHEAT PASTA PLATE OF MIXED GREENS

SERVES 1

2 ounces (50g) buckwheat pasta, cooked by the bundle directions huge bunch of arugula little bunch of basil leaves
8 cherry tomatoes split 1/2 avocado, diced
10 olives

1 tablespoon extra-virgin olive oil 21/2 tablespoons (20g) pine nuts
Tenderly consolidate all the fixings with the exception of the

pine nuts and mastermind on a plate, at that point disperse the pine nuts over the top.

BUCKWHEAT FLAPJACKS WITH STRAWBERRIES, DULL CHOCOLATE SAUCE, AND SQUASHED PECANS

MAKES 6 TO 8 HOTCAKES, CONTINGENT UPON THE SIZE

FOR THE Hotcakes

11/2 cups (350ml) milk

7/8 cup (150g) buckwheat our 1 enormous egg
1 tablespoon extra-virgin olive oil, for cooking

FOR THE CHOCOLATE SAUCE

31/2 ounces (100g) dim chocolate (85 percent cocoa solids) 1/3 cup (85ml) milk

1 tablespoon twofold cream Tablespoon extra-virgin olive oil

TO SERVE

Cups (400g) strawberries, hulled and hacked 7/8 cup (100g) pecans, hacked

To make the flapjack player, place all the fixings separated from the olive oil in a blender and mix until you have a smooth hitter. It ought not to be excessively thick or excessively runny. (You can store any abundance player in an impermeable holder for as long as 5 days in your refrigerator. Make certain to blend a long time before utilizing once more.)

To make the chocolate sauce, liquefy the chocolate in a heatproof bowl over a dish of stewing water. When it's softened, blend in the milk, whisking completely, and afterward include the twofold cream and olive oil. You can keep the sauce warm by leaving the water in the skillet stewing on low warmth until your hotcakes are prepared.

To make the hotcakes, heat a little or medium-size

overwhelming bottomed griddle until it begins to smoke, at that point include the olive oil.

Empty a portion of the hitter into the focal point of the skillet, at that point tip the overabundance player around it until you have secured the entire surface; you may need to add somewhat more player to accomplish this. You will just need to cook the flapjack for 1 moment or so on each side if your dish is sufficiently hot.

When you can see it going earthy colored around the edges, utilize a spatula to extricate the flapjack around its edge, at that point flip it over. Attempt to flip in one activity to abstain from breaking it. Cook for one more moment or so on the opposite side, and move to a plate.

Spot a few strawberries in the inside and move up the flapjack. Proceed until you have made the same number of hotcakes as required.

Spoon a liberal measure of sauce over every hotcake and sprinkle with some slashed pecans.

You may find that your first endeavors are excessively fat or self-destruct, however once you discover the consistency for your hitter that works best for you and you flawless your method, you'll be making them like an expert. Careful discipline brings about promising results for this situation.

TOFU AND SHIITAKE MUSHROOM SOUP

SERVES 4

1/3 ounce (10g) dried (ocean growth) 1 quart (1 liter) vegetable stock

7 ounces (200g) shiitake mushrooms cut 1/3 cup (120g) miso glue

X 14-ounce (400g) square firm tofu, cut into little blocks Scallions, cut and cut on the inclining

1 Thai bean stew, nely slashed (discretionary)

Splash the wakame in warm water for 10 minutes, at that point channel.

Heat the stock to the point of boiling, at that point include the mushrooms and stew delicately for 1 to 2 minutes.
Break down the miso glue in a bowl with a portion of the warm stock to guarantee it disintegrates completely. Add the miso and tofu to the staying stock, taking consideration not to let the soup bubble as this would ruin the fragile miso flavor. Include the depleted wakame, scallions, and bean stew, if utilizing, and serve.

SIRTFOOD CHOMPS

MAKES 15 TO 20 Nibbles 1 cup (120g) pecans
1 ounce (30g) dim chocolate (85 percent cocoa solids), broken into pieces; or 1/4 cup cocoa nibs 9 ounces (250g) Medjool dates, pitted
1 tablespoon cocoa powder

1 tablespoon ground turmeric 1 tablespoon extra-virgin olive oil the scratched seeds of 1 vanilla case or 1 teaspoon vanilla concentrates 1 to 2 tablespoons water
Spot the pecans and chocolate in a food processor and procedure until you have a fine powder. Include the various fixings aside from the water and mix until the blend frames a ball. You might need to include the water depending the consistency of the blend—you don't need it to be excessively clingy.
Utilizing your hands, structure the blend into scaled down balls and refrigerate in a sealed shut holder for at any rate 1 hour before eating them. You could move a portion of the balls in some more cocoa or dried coconut to accomplish an alternate completion on the off chance that you like. They will keep for as long as multi week in your refrigerator.

REFERENCES

SIRTFOOD DIET REFERENCE

☐ Bertie, M. L., et al. "Dietary avonoid admission and weight upkeep: three forthcoming companions of 124,086 US people followed for as long as 24 years." BMJ 352:i17 (2016).

☐ Rabadan-Chávez, G., et al. "Cocoa powder, cocoa extricate, and epicatechin weaken hyper caloric diet-initiated weight through upgraded β-oxidation and vitality consumption in white fat tissue." J Funk Foods 20, 54–67 (2016).

☐ Amphora, A., Maruthappu, M., and Stephenson, T. "Good dieting: a NHS need; a definite method to improve wellbeing results for NHS staff and people in general." Postgrad Med J 90, 671–72 (2014).

☐ Estrus, R., et al. "Essential avoidance of cardiovascular malady with a Mediterranean eating routine." N Engle J Med 368, 1279–90 (2013).

☐ Tresserra-Rimbau, Anna, et al. "Polyphenol admission and mortality chance: a reanalysis of the PREDIMED preliminary." BMC Med 12.1, 1 (2014).

☐ Section 1: THE SCIENCE OF SIRTUINS

☐ Li, X. "SIRT1 and vitality digestion." Act Biochip Biopsy's Sin (Shanghai) 45, 51–60 (2013).

☐ Morris, B. J. "Seven sirtuins for seven fatal maladies of maturing." Free Radica Boil Med 56, 133–71 (2013).

☐ Fontana, L., Partridge, L., and Longo, V. D. "Broadening solid life expectancy — from yeast to people." Science 328, 321–26 (2010).

☐ Ibid.

☐ Haggis, M. C., and Guarantee, L. P. "Mammalian sirtuins—developing jobs in physiology, maturing, and calorie limitation." Genes Dev. 20, 2913–21 (2006).

☐ Radar, Z., et al. "Redox-directing sirtuins in maturing, caloric limitation, and exercise." Free Radica Boil Med 58, 87–97 (2013).

☐ Salinger, J. C., O'Connor, S. M., Wong, J. D., and Don élan, J. M. "People can ceaselessly streamline vivacious expense during strolling." Cur Boil 25, 2452–56 (2015).

☐ Scour, P., O'Keefe, J. H., Marot, J. L., Lange, P., and Jensen, G. B. "Portion of running and long haul mortality: the Copenhagen City Heart Study." J Am Cull Cardio 65, 411–19 (2015).

☐ Mons, U., Haman, H., and Brenner, H. "A converse J-formed relationship of recreation time physical movement with visualization in patients with stable coronary illness: proof from a huge companion with rehashed estimations." Heart 100, 1043–49 (2014).

SECTION 2: FIGHTING FAT

☐ Burdon, L., et al. "SIRT1 transgenic mice show phenotypes taking after calorie limitation." Aging Cell 6, 759–67 (2007).

☐ Chalkiadaki, An., and Guarantee, L. "High-fat eating routine triggers in ammationinduced cleavage of SIRT1 in fat tissue to advance metabolic brokenness." Cell Metal 16, 180–88 (2012).

☐ Costa Cods, S., et al. "SIRT1 interpretation is diminished in instinctive fat tissue of butterball shaped patients with extreme hepatic statuses." Obese Surge 20, 633–39 (2010).

☐ Pedersen, S. B., Loom, J., Paulsen, S. K., Bentsen, M. F., and Michelson, B. "Low SIRT1 articulation, which is up regulated by fasting, in human fat tissue from stout ladies." Into J Obese (Lund) 32, 1250–55 (2008).

☐ Milliken's, M. C., et al. "SIRT1 hereditary variety is identified with BMI and danger of stoutness." Diabetes 58, 2828–34 (2009).

Tontines, P., and Spiegel man, B. M. "Fat and past: the assorted science of PPARgamma." Annu Rev Brioche 77, 289–312 (2008).

Picard, F., et al. "SIRT1 advances fat assembly in white adipocytes by stifling PPAR-gamma." Nature 429, 771–76 (2004).

Qing, L., et al. "Earthy colored renovating of white fat tissue by SIRT1dependent DE acetylation of Ppargamma." Cell 150, 620–32 (2012).

Li, X. "SIRT1 and vitality digestion." Act Biochip Biopsy's Sin (Shanghai) 45, 51–60 (2013).

Akieda-Asai, S., et al. "SIRT1 manages thyroid-animating hormone discharge by improving PIP5Kgamma action through DE acetylation of specie c lysine buildups in vertebrates." Plops One 5, e11755 (2010).

Aragon's, G., et al. "Balance of leptin opposition by food mixes." Moll Nut Food Res 60, 1789–803 (2016).

Sasaki, T. "Age-related weight gain, leptin, and SIRT1: a potential job for hypothalamic SIRT1 in the avoidance of weight increase and maturing through regulation of leptin affectability." Front Endocrinal 6, 109 (2015).

SECTION 3: MASTERS OF MUSCLE

Audile, L. Z., et al. "Skeletal muscle PGC-1alpha1 regulates kynurenine digestion and intercedes flexibility to push actuated discouragement." Cell 159, 33–45 (2014).

Sharples, A. P., et al. "Life span and skeletal bulk: the job of IGF flagging, the sirtuins, dietary limitation, and protein admission." Aging Cell 14, 511–23 (2015).

Diaz-Ruiz, A., Gonzalez-Freire, M., Verruca, L., Bernier, M., and de Cabot, R. "SIRT1 synchronizes satellite cell digestion with undifferentiated cell destiny." Cell Stem Cell 16, 103–4 (2015).

☐ Rathbone, C. R., Booth, F. W., and Lees, S. J. "SIRT1 increments skeletal muscle forerunner cell expansion." Ear J Cell Boil 88, 35–44 (2009).

☐ Lee, D., and Goldberg, A. L. "SIRT1 protein, by obstructing the exercises of translation factors FoxO1 and FoxO3, hinders muscle decay and advances muscle development." J Boil CChem 288, 30515–26 (2013).

☐ Royall, J. G., et al. "The NAD(+)- subordinate SIRT1 deacetylase makes an interpretation of a metabolic switch into administrative epigenetics in skeletal muscle immature microorganisms." Cell Stem Cell 16, 171–83 (2015).

☐ Lee and Goldberg. "SIRT1 protein."

☐ Sharples. "Life span and skeletal bulk."

☐ Lee and Goldberg. "SIRT1 protein."

☐ In the same place.

☐ Sharples. "Life span and skeletal bulk."

☐ Sousa-Victor, P., García-Prat, L., Serrano, A. L., Perdiguero, E., and Muñoz-Canoes, P. "Muscle immature microorganism maturing: guideline and revival." Trends Endocrinal Metal 26, 287– 96 (2015).

☐ Tonkin, J., Villarreal, F., Pure, P. L., and Vinci Guerra, M. "SIRT1 motioning as potential modulator of skeletal muscle sicknesses." Cur Open Pharmacology 12, 372–76 (2012).

☐ Rebase, M., et al. "Relationship between both absolute gauge urinary and dietary polyphenols and considerable physical execution decrease chance in more seasoned grown- ups: a 9-year follow-up of the In CHIANTI study." J Nutria Health Aging 20.5, 478–84 (2016).

☐ Cohen, S., Nathan, J. An., and Goldberg, A. L. "Muscle squandering in malady: sub-atomic instruments and promising treatments." Nat Rev Drug Disco 14, 58–74 (2015).

SECTION 4: WELL-BEING WONDERS

☐ Ma, L., and Li, Y. "SIRT1: job in cardiovascular science." Clan Chime Act 440, 8–15 (2015).

☐ Ibid.

☐ Milne, J. C., et al. "Little atom activators of SIRT1 as therapeutics for the treatment of type 2 diabetes." Nature 450, 712–16 (2007).

☐ Fu, L., et al. "Leucine ample as the impacts of metformin on insulin affectability and glycemic control in diet-incited fat mice." Metabolism 64, 845–56 (2015).

☐ Wang, J., et al. "The job of SIRT1: at the junction between advancement of life span and insurance against Alzheimer's ailment neuropathology." Biochip Biopsy's Act 1804, 1690–94 (2010).

☐ Goblin, W., Skinner, M. E., and Lombard, D. B. "Sirtuins: watchmen of mammalian health span." Trends Genet 30, 271–86 (2014).

☐ Ayer, S., et al. "Sirtuin1 (SIRT1) advances cortical bone arrangement by forestalling beta- catenin sequestration by Fox translation factors in osteoblast ancestors." J Boil CChem 289, 24069–78 (2014).

☐ Walking, M. J., and Ahmad, N. "The job of SIRT1 in disease: the adventure proceeds." Is J Pathos 185, 26–28 (2015).

SECTION 5: SIRTFOODS

☐ Weitzman, M. F., et al. "Physical action proposals and diminished danger of mortality." Arch Intern Med 167, 2453–60 (2007).

☐ Kennedy, D. O. "Polyphenols and the human mind: plant 'auxiliary metabolite' ecologic jobs and endogenous flagging capacities drive benefits." Adv. Nutria 5, 515–33 (2014).

☐ Hooper, P. L., Hooper, P. L., Tyrell, M., and Vigo, L. "Xenohormesis: medical advantages from an age of plant pressure reaction advancement." Cell Stress Chaperones 15, 761–70 (2010).

☐ Ibid.

☐ Howitz, K. T., and Sinclair, D. A. "Xenohormesis: detecting the substance signs of different species." Cell 133, 387–91 (2008).

☐ Howitz, K. T., et al. "Little atom activators of sirtuins broaden Saccharomyces cerevisiae life expectancy." Nature 425, 191–96 (2003).

☐ Madeo, F., Pietrocola, F., Eisenberg, T., and Kroemer, G. "Caloric limitation mimetic: towards an atomic de nation." Nat Rev Drug Disco 13, 727–40 (2014).

☐ Bonkowski and Sinclair. "Easing back maturing by plan."

☐ Chung, S., et al. "Guideline of SIRT1 in cell capacities: job of polyphenols." Arch Brioche Biopsy's 501, 79–90 (2010).

☐ Howitz, et al. "Little atom activators of sirtuins."

☐ Si, H., and Liu, D. "Dietary anticaking phytochemicals and components related with delayed endurance." J Nutria Brioche 25, 581–91 (2014).

☐ Xiao, N., et al. "Quercetin, lutein, and epigallocatechin gallate advance glucose removal in adipocytes with guideline of AMP-initiated kinase and additionally sirtuin 1 action." Plantae Med 80, 993–1000 (2014).

☐ Putsch, K. "Chromatins, cancer prevention agents and prooxidants: de nine quercetin-, coffee corrosive and rosmarinic corrosive interceded life expansion in C. elegant." Bio gerontology 12, 329–47 (2011).

☐ Vanilla, L., et al. "Coffee corrosive phenethyl ester controls PPAR's levels in undifferentiated cells inferred adipocytes." PPAR Research (2016).

☐ Scanned, C., et al. "Flavonoid apigenin is an inhibitor of the

NAD+ as CD38: suggestions for cell NAD+ digestion, protein acetylation, and treatment of metabolic disorder." Diabetes 4, 1084–93 (2013).

☐ Rabadan-Chávez, et al. "Cocoa powder, cocoa separate, and epicatechin."

☐ Duarte, D. An., et al. "Polyphenol-improved cocoa shields the diabetic retina from glial response through the sirtuin pathway." J Nutria Brioche 26, 64–74 (2015).

☐ Ramirez-Sanchez, I., et al. "(-)- Epicatechin rich cocoa intervened balance of oxidative pressure controllers in skeletal muscle of cardiovascular breakdown and type 2 diabetes patients." Into J Cardio 168, 3982–90 (2013).

☐ Ye, Q. "Epigallocatechin-3-gallate smothers 1-methyl-4-phenyl-pyridineinduced oxidative worry in PC12 cells through the SIRT1/PGC-1α flagging pathway." BMC Complement Alter Med 12, 82 (2012).

☐ Lee, M. S., et al. "Green tea (-)- epigallotocatechin-3-gallate prompts PGC1α quality articulation in HepG2 cells and 3T3-L1 adipocytes." Prep Nutria Food Sic 1, 62–67 (2016).

☐ Zhang, X., et al. "Dietary lutein actuates searing and thermogenesis in mice through an AMPK/PGC1α pathway-interceded component." Into J Obese (Lund) (2016).

☐ Dong, J., et al. "Quercetin lessens corpulence related ATM in alteration and in ambition in mice: a system including AMPKα1/SIRT1." J Lipid Res 55, 363–74 (2014).

☐ Davis, J. M. "Quercetin builds mind and muscle mitochondrial biogenesis and exercise resistance." Am J Physiology Regal Integer Comp Physiology 296, 1071–77 (2009).

☐ Su, K. Y., et al. "Rutin, an avonoid and head part of saussurea involucrate, constricts physical exhaustion in a constrained swimming mouse model." Into J Med Sic 11, 528–37 (2014).

☐ Goo, Z. "Kaempferol secures cardiomyocytes against anoxia/oxygenation injury by means of mitochondrial pathway interceded by SIRT1." Ear J Pharmacology 761, 245–53c (2015).

Menendez, J. An., et al. "Xenohormetic and hostile to maturing movement of secoiridoid polyphenols present in additional virgin olive oil: another group of gerosuppressant operators." Cell Cycle 12, 555–78 (2013).

Kikusato, M., et al. "Oleuropein prompts mitochondrial biogenesis and diminishes responsive oxygen species age in refined avian muscle cells, perhaps through an up- guideline of peroxisome proliferator-initiated receptor γ coactivator1α." Amin Sic J (2016).

Luccarini, I., et al. "The polyphenol oleuropein glycine tweaks the PARP1-SIRT1 exchange: an in vitro and in vivo examination." J Alzheimer's Dis (2016).

Sheng, An., et al. "Hydroxytyrosol improves mitochondrial work and decreases oxidative worry in the cerebrum of dB/dB mice: job of AMP-initiated protein kinase actuation." Br J Nutria 113, 1667–76 (2015).

Doan, Khan V., et al. "Gallic corrosive directs body weight and glucose homeostasis through AMPK enactment." Endocrinology 156, 157–68 (2014).

Rabat, K. An., and Schnellmann, R. G. "Iso avones advance mitochondrial biogenesis." J Pharmacology Exp Ther 325, 536–43 (2008).

Hong, K. S. "Contribution of SIRT1 in hypoxic down-guideline of c-Myc and β-catenin and hypoxic preconditioning impact of polyphenols." Toxically Apple Pharmacology 259, 210–8 (2012).

Yama, K. D., and Chaudhary, A. K. "Hostile to corpulence system of Curcuma longa L.: a diagram." IJNPR-in the past NPR 7, 99–106 (2016).

Lee, M. S., et al. "Decrease of body weight by dietary garlic is related with an expansion in uncoupling protein mRNA articulation and enactment of AMP-actuated protein kinase in diet-prompted stout mice." J Nutria 141, 1947–53 (2011).

Jin, T. "Fisting up-controls the statement of adiponectin in 3T3-L1 adipocytes through the enactment of quiet mating type data guideline 2 homologue 1 (SIRT1)- deacetylase and peroxisome proliferator-actuated receptors (PPARs)." J Agaric Food CChem 62, 10468–74 (2014).

SECTION 6: SIRTFOODS AROUND THE WORLD

Bayard, V., Chamorro, F., Motta, J., and Hollinger, N. K. "Does avanol consumption in hence mortality from nitric oxide–subordinate procedures? Ischemic coronary illness, stroke, diabetes mellitus, and disease in Panama." Into J Med Sic 4, 53–58 (2007).

Shrike, M. G., et al. "Flavonoid-rich cocoa utilization influences numerous cardiovascular hazard factors in a meta-investigation of momentary examinations." J Nutria 141, 1982–88 (2011).

Hooper, L., et al. "Impacts of chocolate, cocoa, and avan-3-ols on cardiovascular wellbeing: an orderly survey and meta-investigation of randomized preliminaries." Am J Clan Nutria 95, 740–51 (2012).

Duarte, D. An., et al. "Polyphenol-advanced cocoa secures the diabetic retina."

Martin, M. A., Goya, L., and Ramos, S. "Potential for preventive impacts of cocoa and cocoa polyphenols in malignancy." Food CChem Toxically 56, 336–51 (2013).

Brickman, A. M., et al. "Upgrading dentate gyros work with dietary avanols improves cognizance in more seasoned grown-ups." Nat Neurosis 17, 1798–803 (2014).

Verrazano, G. F., et al. "Hostile to cariogenic impacts of polyphenols from plant energizer drinks (cocoa, espresso, tea)." Fitoterapia 8, 255–62 (2009).

Hutchins-Wolf Brandt, An., and Misty, A. M. "Dietary turmeric possibly diminishes the danger of malignant growth." Asian Pac J Cancer Prep 12, 3169–73 (2011).

Panache, Y., et al. "Cancer prevention agent and hostile to in amatory impacts of curcuminoid-piperine blend in subjects with metabolic condition: a randomized controlled preliminary and a refreshed meta-examination." Clan Nutria (2015).

☐ Kuptniratsaikul, V., Thanakhumtorn, S., Chinswang-watanakul, P., Wattanamongkonsil, L., and Thamlikitkul, V. "Ef cay and security of Curcuma domestic removes in patients with knee osteoarthritis." J Alter Complement Med 15, 891–97 (2009).

☐ Yama and Chaudhary. "Hostile to heftiness instrument of Curcuma longa L."

☐ Lee, M. S., et al. "Turmeric improves post-prandial working memory in pre-diabetes free of insulin." Asia Pac J Clan Nutria 23, 581–91 (2014).

☐ So , F., Cesar, F., Abate, R., Gemini, G. F., and Cassini, A. "Adherence to Mediterranean eating routine and wellbeing status: meta-examination." BMJ 11, 337:a1344 (2008).

☐ Naquin, C., et al. "The Mediterranean eating routine secures against abdomen boundary extension in 12Ala bearers for the PPARgamma quality: 2 years' follow-up of 774 subjects at high cardiovascular hazard." Br J Nutria 102, 672–79 (2009).

☐ Ibarrola-Jurado, N., et al. "Cross-sectional evaluation of nut utilization and heftiness, metabolic condition and other cardio metabolic hazard factors:

☐ The PREDIMED study." Plops One 8, e57367 (2013).

SECTION 7: BUILDING A DIET THAT WORKS

☐ Hertzog, M. G., et al. "Flavonoid consumption and long haul danger of coronary illness and disease in the seven nations study." Arch Intern Med 155, 381–86 (1995).

☐ Ibid.

☐ Bilge, M., and Borelli, A. A. "Wine, liquor and pills: what future for the French conundrum?" Life Sic 131, 19–22 (2015).

☐ Orton, J., et al. "Network impacts on the bioavailability of resveratrol in people." Food CChem 120, 1123–30 (2010).

Gupta, Sub ash C., et al. "Curcumin, a part of turmeric: from homestead to drug store." Bio factors 39, 2–13 (2013).

Elsberry, I., Miranda, J., Lassa, A., Churros, I., and Portillo, M. P. "Dosages of quercetin in the scope of serum fixations apply dilapidating impacts in 3T3-L1 preadipocytes by following up on various phases of abiogenesis, however not in develop adipocytes." Oxide Med Cell Longed 2015, 480943 (2015).

Steepens, A., Tan, K., and Paxton, J. W. "Improving the oral bioavailability of been coal polyphenols through planned cooperative energies." Genes Nutria 5, 75–87 (2010).

Bohn, T. "Dietary variables influencing polyphenol bioavailability." Nutria Rev 72, 429–52 (2014).

Yu, Y., et al. "Green tea catechins: a new aver to anticancer treatment." Apoptosis 19, 1–18 (2014).

Bohn, "Dietary components influencing polyphenol bioavailability."

Yao, K., Duane, Y., Tan, B., Hour, Y., Wu, G., and Yin, Y. "Leucine in weight: helpful possibilities." Trends Pharmacology Sic 8 (2016).

Bruckbauer, An., and Zexel, M. B. "Synergistic impacts of polyphenols and methylxanthines with Leucine on AMPK/Sirtuin-interceded digestion in muscle cells and adipocytes." Plops One 9, e89166 (2014).

Feldman, J. L., Baez, J., and Danu, J. M. "Actuation of the protein deacetylase SIRT6 by long- chain unsaturated fats and boundless DE acylation by mammalian sirtuins." J Boil CChem 288, 31350–56 (2013).

Attunes, L. C., Levandovski, R., Danas, G., Cuomo, W., and Hidalgo, M. P. "Weight and move work: chronobiological perspectives." Nutria Res Rev 23, 155–68 (2010).

Pan, A., Schernhammer, E. S., Sun, Q., and Hu, F. B. "Turning night move work and danger of type 2 diabetes: two forthcoming accomplice concentrates in ladies." Plops Med 8, e1001141 (2011).

☐ Ribas-Latre, An., and Deckle-Mahan, K. "Association of supplement digestion and the circadian clock framework: significance for metabolic wellbeing." Moll Metal 5, 133–52 (2016).

☐ Wegner, D. M., Schneider, D. J., Carter, S. R. third, and White, T. L. "Incomprehensible impacts of thought concealment." J Peers Sock Psyche 53, 5–13 (1987).

SECTION 8: TOP TWENTY SIRTFOODS

☐ Bastian, B., Jetton, J., and Ferris, L. J. "Agony as social paste: shared torment expands collaboration." Psyche Sic 25, 2079–85 (2014).

☐ Live, J., et al. "Utilization of hot nourishments and aggregate and cause specie c mortality: populace based associate investigation." BMJ 351, h3942 (2015).

☐ Ding, M., Bhupathiraju, S. N., Chen, M., van Dam, R. M., and Hu, F. B. "Energized and decaffeinated espresso utilization and danger of type 2 diabetes: an orderly audit and a portion reaction meta-examination." Diabetes Care 37, 569–86 (2014).

☐ Bohn, S. K., Blomhoff, R., and Pair, I. "Espresso and malignant growth chance, epidemiological proof, and sub-atomic systems." Moll Nutria Food Res 58, 915–30 (2014).

☐ Wirdefeldt, K., Adam, H. O., Cole, P., Trichopoulos, D., and Mandel, J. "The study of disease transmission and etiology of Parkinson's illness: a survey of the proof." Ear J Epidemiology 26 Supple 1, S1–58 (2011).

☐ Master ton, G. S., and Hayes, P. C. "Espresso and the liver: a potential treatment for liver illness?" Ear J Gastroenterology Hepatic 22, 1277–83 (2010).

☐ Hussein, An., and Hosseinzadeh, H. "An audit on the impacts of Allium sativa (Garlic) in metabolic condition." J Endocrinal Invest 38, 1147–157 (2015).

☐ Failover, J., Roberts, S. C., and Havelock, J. "Utilization of garlic decidedly influences epicurean impression of axillary personal stench." Appetite 97, 8–15 (2016).

☐ Alkali, J. M., et al. "Glycemic files of vet assortments of dates in sound and diabetic subjects." Nutria J 10, 59 (2011).

☐ Avail, P. K. "Date organic products (Phoenix dactylifera Linn): a rising restorative food." Crist Rev Food Sic Nutria 52, 249–71 (2012).

☐ Beluga, M. S., Beluga, B. R. V., Kandathil, S. M., Bhatt, H. P., and Avail, P. K. "An audit of the science and pharmacology of the date natural products (Phoenix dactylifera L.)." Food Res into 44, 1812–22 (2011).

☐ Takkouche, B., et al. "Admission of wine, brew, and spirits and the danger of clinical regular virus." Am J Epidemiology 155, 853–58 (2002).

☐ Muñoz-González, I., Thornier, T., Bartolommeo, B., and Moreno-Arriba's, M. V. "Red wine and oenological removes show antimicrobial impacts in an oral microscopic organisms bio lm model." J Agaric Food CChem 62, 4731–37 (2014).

☐ Torreon, R., et al. "Berries decrease postprandial insulin reactions to wheat and rye breads in solid ladies." J Nutria 143, 430–36 (2013).

SECTION 9: PHASE 1: 7 POUNDS IN SEVEN DAYS

☐ Nestea, T., et al. "Bioactive creation and cell reinforcement capability of various normally expended espresso blends influenced by their arrangement procedure and milk expansion." Food CChem 134, 1870–77 (2012).

☐ Hurtle, R., and Westerterp-Plantenga, M. S. "Utilization of milk protein joined with green tea balances diet-initiated thermogenesis." Nutrients 3, 725–33 (2011).

☐ Green, R. J., Murphy, A. S., Schulz, B., Watkins, B. An., and Peruzzi, M. G. "Normal tea plans adjust in vitro stomach related recuperation of green tea catechins." Moll Nutria Food Res 51, 1152–62 (2007).

SECTION 10: SIRTFOODS FOR LIFE

Malik, B. C. "Milk—a supplement arrangement of mammalian advancement advancing mTORC1-subordinate interpretation." Into J Moll Sic 16, 17048–87 (2015).

Liu, M., et al. "Resveratrol hinders motor motioning by advancing the collaboration among motor and DEPTOR." J Boil CChem 285, 36387–94

(2010).

Aunt, D., et al. "Dairy items and colorectal malignant growth hazard: a methodical survey and meta-examination of associate investigations." Ann Uncool 23, 37–45 (2012).

Aunt, D., et al. "Dairy items, calcium, and prostate disease chance: a precise audit and meta- investigation of partner examines." Is J Clan Nutria 101, 87–117 (2015).

Devoid, H., Ismailia, S., and Mortazavian, A. "Impacts of milk and milk items utilization on malignancy: an audit." Compr Rev Food Sic Food Saf 12, 249–64 (2013).

Wiseman, M. "The second World Cancer Research Fund/American Institute for Cancer Research master report. Food, sustenance, physical action, and the avoidance of malignant growth: a worldwide viewpoint." Pros Nutria Sock 67, 253–56 (2008).

Person, E., Grazing, G., Ferracane, R., Fogliano, V., and Skog, K. "In hence of cell reinforcements in virgin olive oil on the arrangement of heterocyclic amines in singed beef burgers." Food CChem Toxically 41, 1587–97 (2003).

Gibes, M. "Impact of oil marinades with garlic, onion, and lemon squeeze on the arrangement of heterocyclic sweet-smelling amines in singed hamburger patties." J Agaric Food CChem 55, 10240–47 (2007).

Rohr Mann, S., Hermann, S., and Linseisen, J. "Heterocyclic sweet-smelling amine admission increments colorectal adenoma chance: endings from a forthcoming European accomplice study." Is J Clan Nutria 89, 1418–24 (2009).

Nerurkar, P. V., Le Marchland, L., and Cooney, R. V. "Impacts of marinating with Asian marinades or western grill sauce on Phips and Mix development in grilled hamburger." Nutria Cancer 34, 147–52 (1999).

Rung, Y., et al. "Egg utilization and danger of coronary illness and stroke: portion reaction meta-investigation of imminent accomplice contemplates." BMJ 346, e8539 (2013).

Craig, W. J., Mangles, A. R., and American Dietetic Association. "Position of the American Dietetic Association: vegan slims down." J Am Diet Asoka 109, 1266–82 (2009).

Appleby, P., Rod dam, An., Allen, N., and Key, T. "Relative crack hazard in veggie lovers and non-vegetarians in EPIC-Oxford." Ear J Clan Nutria 61, 1400–1406 (2007).

Krajcovicova-Kudlackova, M., Buck ova, K., Climes, I., and Sebokova, E. "Iodine de cogency in veggie lovers and vegetarians." Ann Nutria Metal 47, 183–85 (2003).

www.ingramcontent.com/pod-product-compliance
Lightning Source LLC
Chambersburg PA
CBHW020917160726

47993CB00005B/2018